# Seniors Illustrated
# Volume 2

Stories by Hank Bruce
Illustrations by Sally Lamas
Poetry & editing by Tomi Jill Folk

Petals & Pages Press
Rio Rancho, New Mexico

# Seniors Illustrated, Volume 2

This is the second in a series of books written expressly with senior readers in mind.



Petals & Pages Press
860 Polaris Blvd SE
Rio Rancho, NM 87124

www.petalsandpagespress.com
petals_pages@msn.com

Published by Petals & Pages Press © 2009

ISBN 978-0-9797057-6-2

Written by Hank Bruce
Illustration by Sally Lamas
Poetry & editing by Tomi Jill Folk

# Seniors Illustrated, Volume 2

## Table of contents:



## More books in this series

*Seniors Illustrated, Vol. 1*
*Barefoot in the Grass* - Flo & Claire conspire to beat the system at Whispering Winds Senior Center. You're invited to join them.
*Fisherman, Fisherman* - an elderly gentleman teaches a wayward youth how to fish.

*Seniors Illustrated, Vol. 3 Special for the Holiday Season*
*For the Love of Luminita* - Thoughtful and thought provoking look at the Christmas story
*Gingerbread Friends* - an intergenerational gingerbread adventure that you can make come true

*Seniors Illustrated, Vol. 4*
*The Gifts* - A Native American elder shares a story about the gift each of us is.
*A Bouquet of Friends* - An elderly lady finds a way to pay tribute to loved ones.

# Eventide

Cattle graze ‘neath the setting sun;

Soon, they’ll rest.  The day is done.

Gentle rays caress the land;

All are safe within God’s hands.

By Tomi Jill Folk

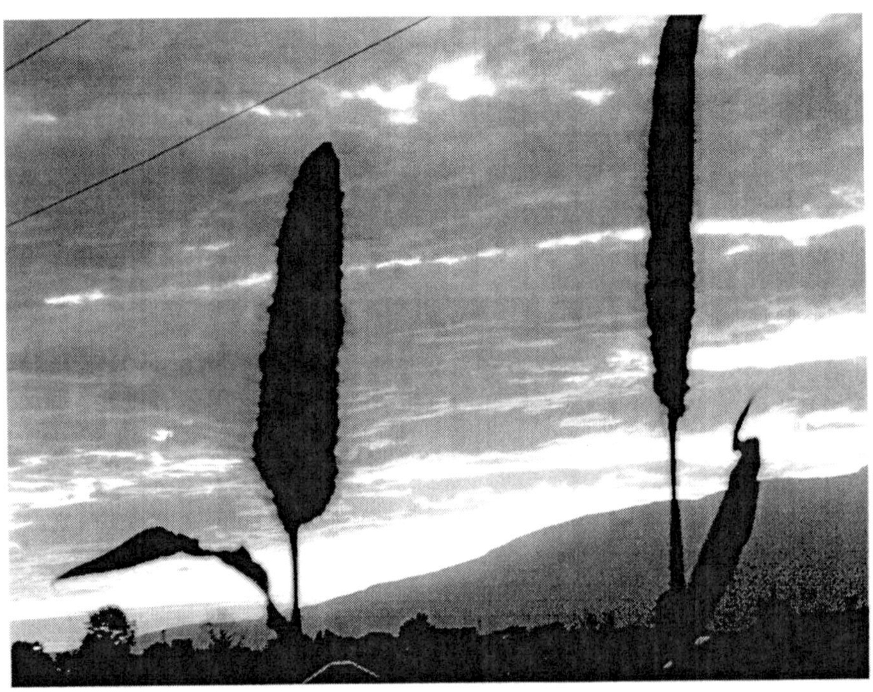

# Cactus Flowers and Friends

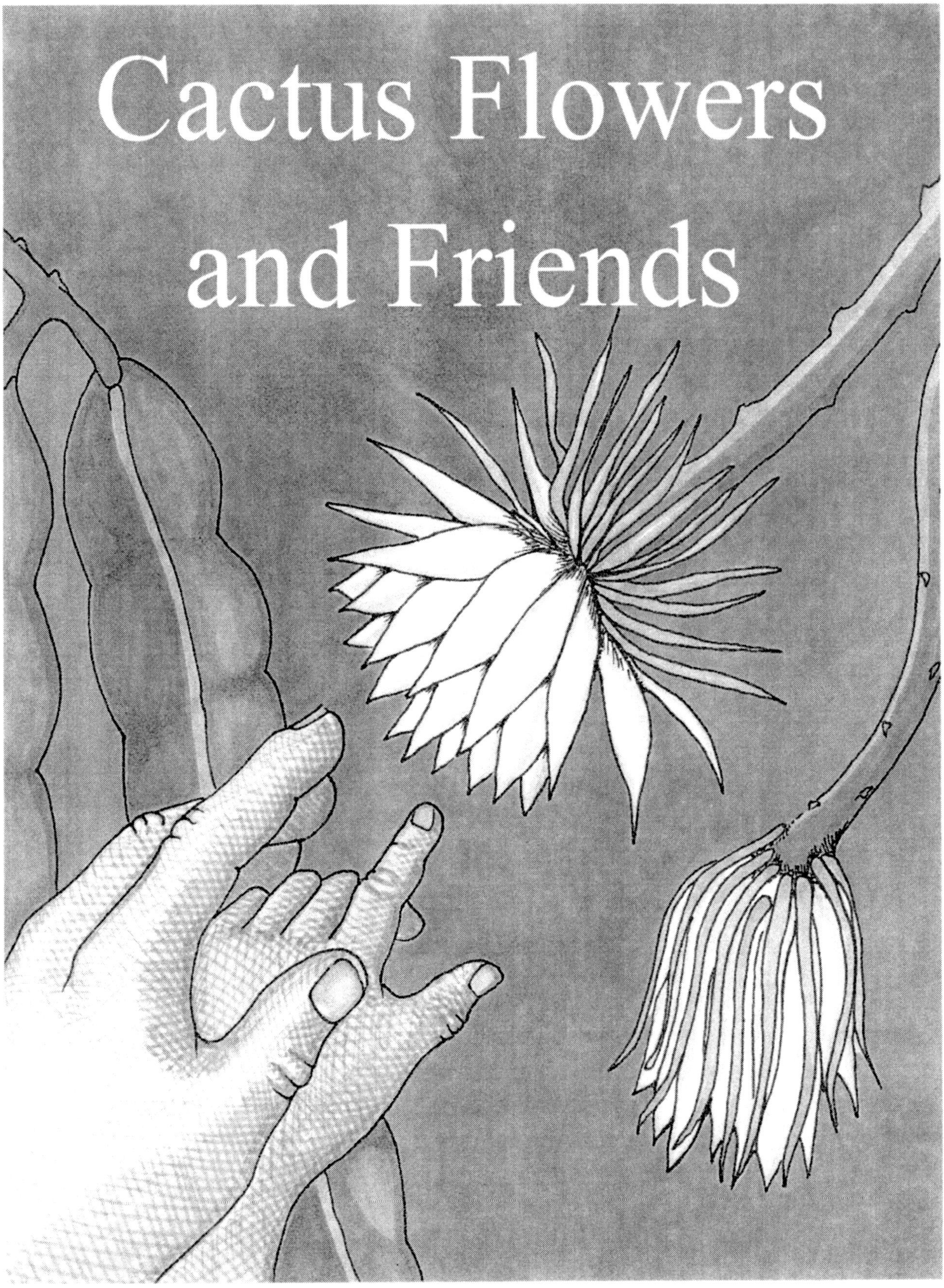

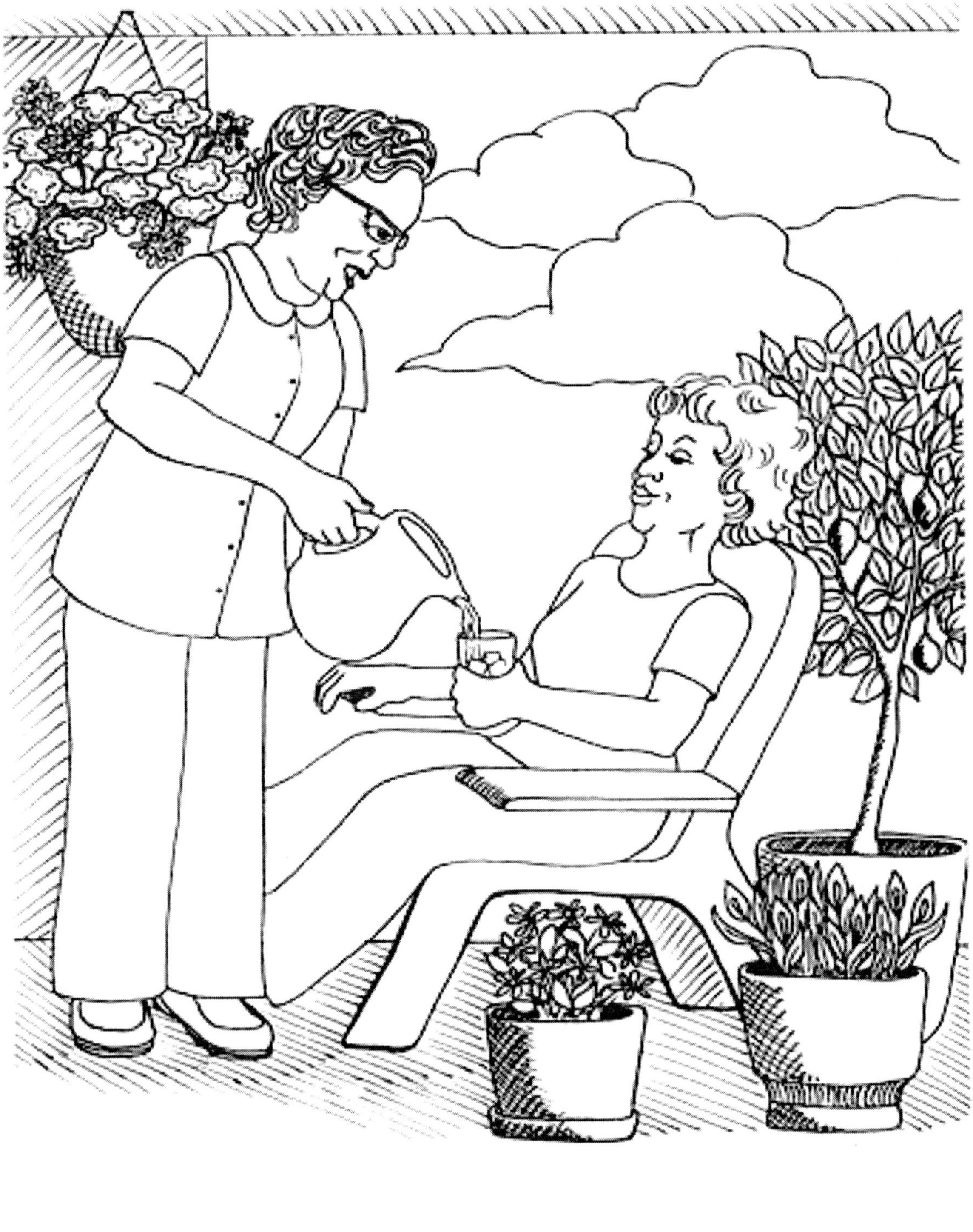

# Cactus Flowers and Friends

by Hank Bruce

It was a hot afternoon in July 1958. Dark clouds had started forming on the horizon.

"Looks like a promise of rain," she said as she refilled the glasses and sat the pitcher of fresh squeezed lemonade on the porch table. All her friends knew her as Billie, but her name was really Wilhelmina.

Dottie was Billie's next door neighbor and best friend. She was studying the plants that surrounded her. Billie had hanging baskets, an avocado that was taller than she was, and a lemon tree that had bloomed in May and now had over a dozen small fruit growing on its thorny branches. Not bad for a back porch in western Pennsylvania.

Billie's green thumb was the talk of the neighborhood. Dottie told everyone the story about Billie being such a good gardener that she could stick a toothpick in a flowerpot and it would grow.

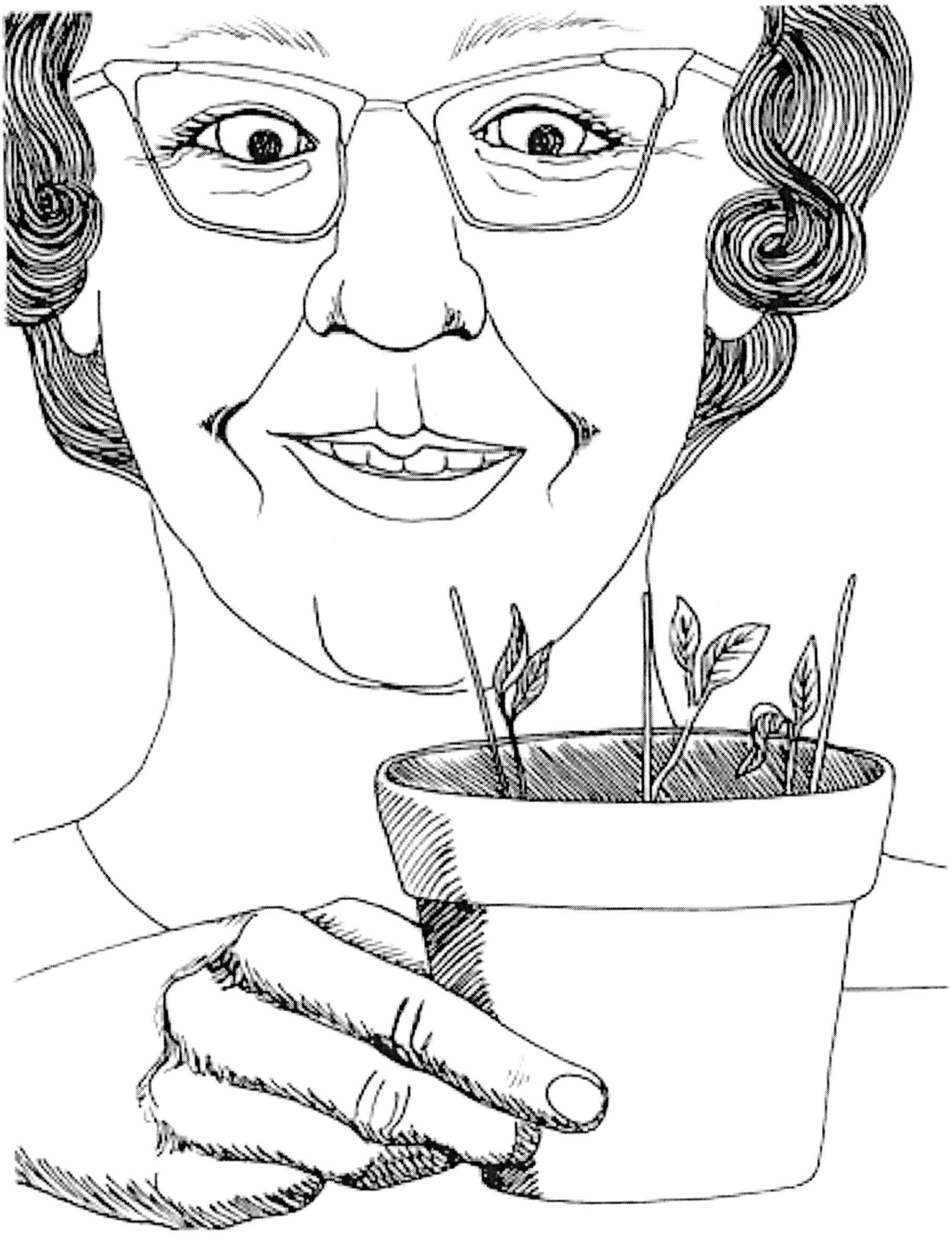

This all started several Christmases ago when Billie had been given the gift of some dates. These dates still had the pits in them.

After she had eaten several of these dates, she stuck the seeds in a flower pot and put it on the windowsill. Then to remind herself of the fact that she had planted seeds in this pot, she stuck a couple toothpicks in the soil next to the seeds.

She kept it watered, and in February the first of the seeds sprouted. Her son, as a joke, told everyone it was the toothpick that had taken root and now sported a large new leaf. Some took his joke seriously and the story spread about Billie sprouting toothpicks.

Now Dottie and Billie were planning a party. Billie slowly walked over to the large hanging basket that hung from the corner of this porch.

"This old cactus has gotta be the ugliest plant I've got," she said as she carefully touched the thick green stems. Some were wrapped around the wires while others draped down. There were a few spines, but with a little caution they could be avoided.

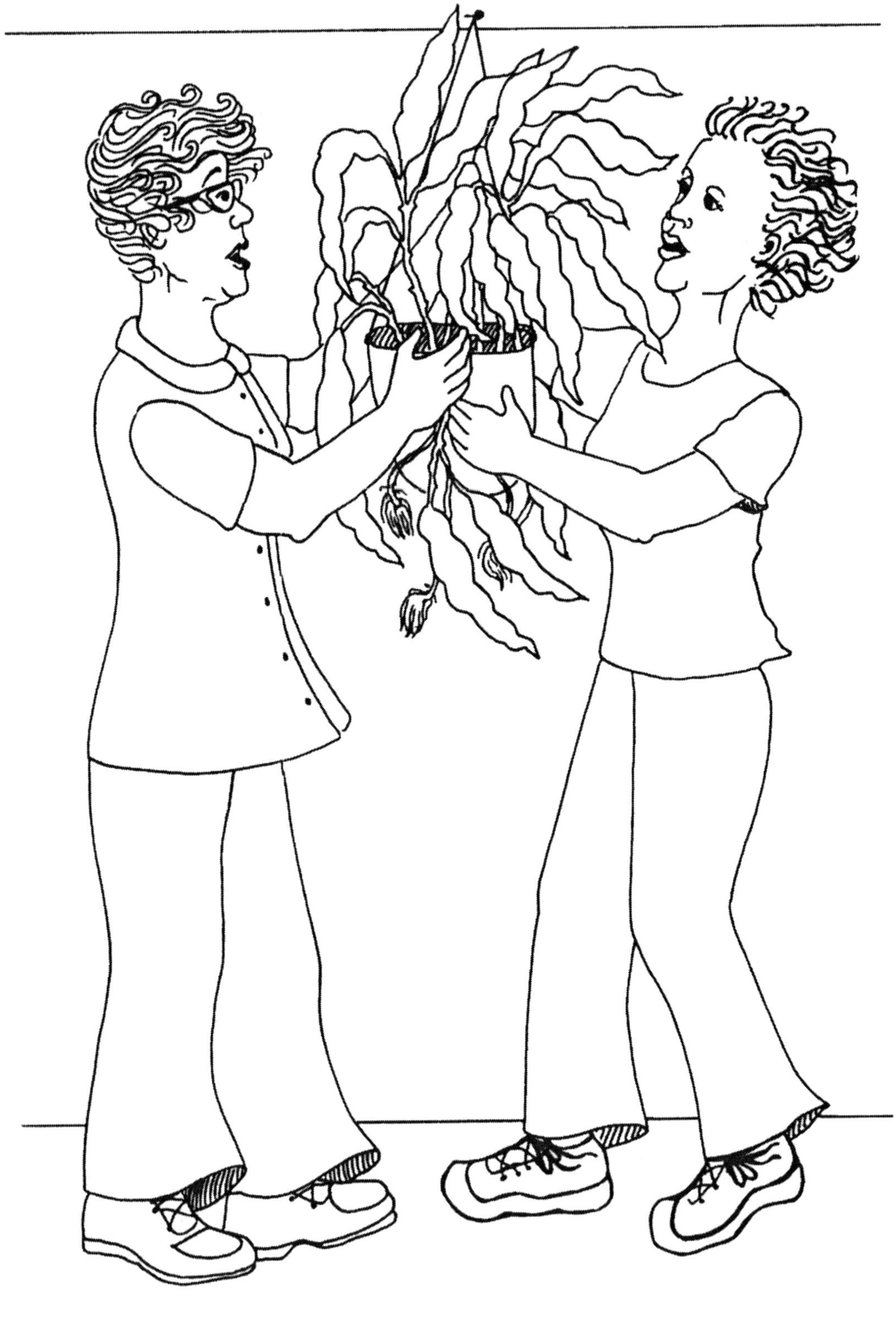

Dottie joined her friend just as the first distant rumble of thunder was heard. The wind came next. It was so strong that the hanging basket with the ivy geranium started swinging.

The lightning flashed and the second gust of wind hit them hard. The geranium basket came smashing down onto the wooden porch floor.

The two ladies grabbed the huge cactus just as the wind set it swinging. After all, this plant was the reason for the party. It was the guest of honor. This was a special year because this time the night blooming cereus had three buds.

Perhaps you have never seen a night blooming cereus bloom. It slowly opens its snow white flowers in the darkness of a moonless night. It is one of the truly amazing sights the plant world has to offer.

Billie had nursed and nurtured this plant for over six years.

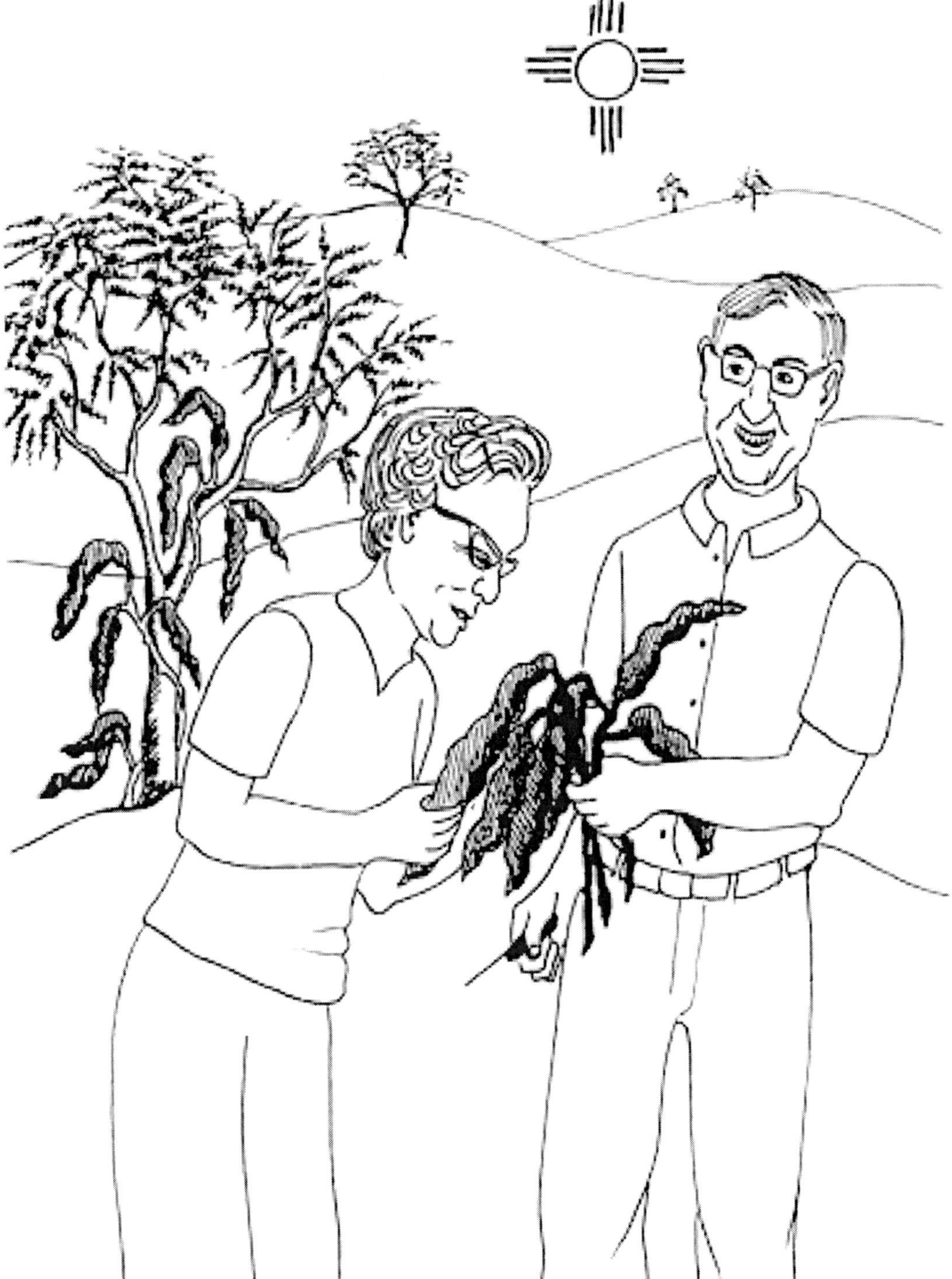

Six years ago Billie and Purdy had been on a vacation that took them through southern New Mexico, almost to the Mexican border. At a roadside rest they had stopped to let the old Chevy station wagon cool off while they shared a picnic lunch.

Purdy saw the strange looking cactus twining up the mesquite trees in the desert that spread out before them. He took a piece of newspaper and his pocket knife and walked over to investigate.

He returned with three cuttings. After showing them to Billie, they were wrapped in the newspaper and tucked under the seat of the old "Woody."

Billie had no idea what this weird cactus plant was, but, when they returned home, she stuck the three cuttings in an old Chase & Sanborn coffee can Purdy had filled with soil. These ugly cactus cuttings sat on the corner of the porch through the summer.

It wasn't until she began moving the plants indoors for the winter that she rediscovered this ugly excuse for a cactus. The cuttings had taken root. A couple new branches had formed and it seemed to be thriving on neglect.

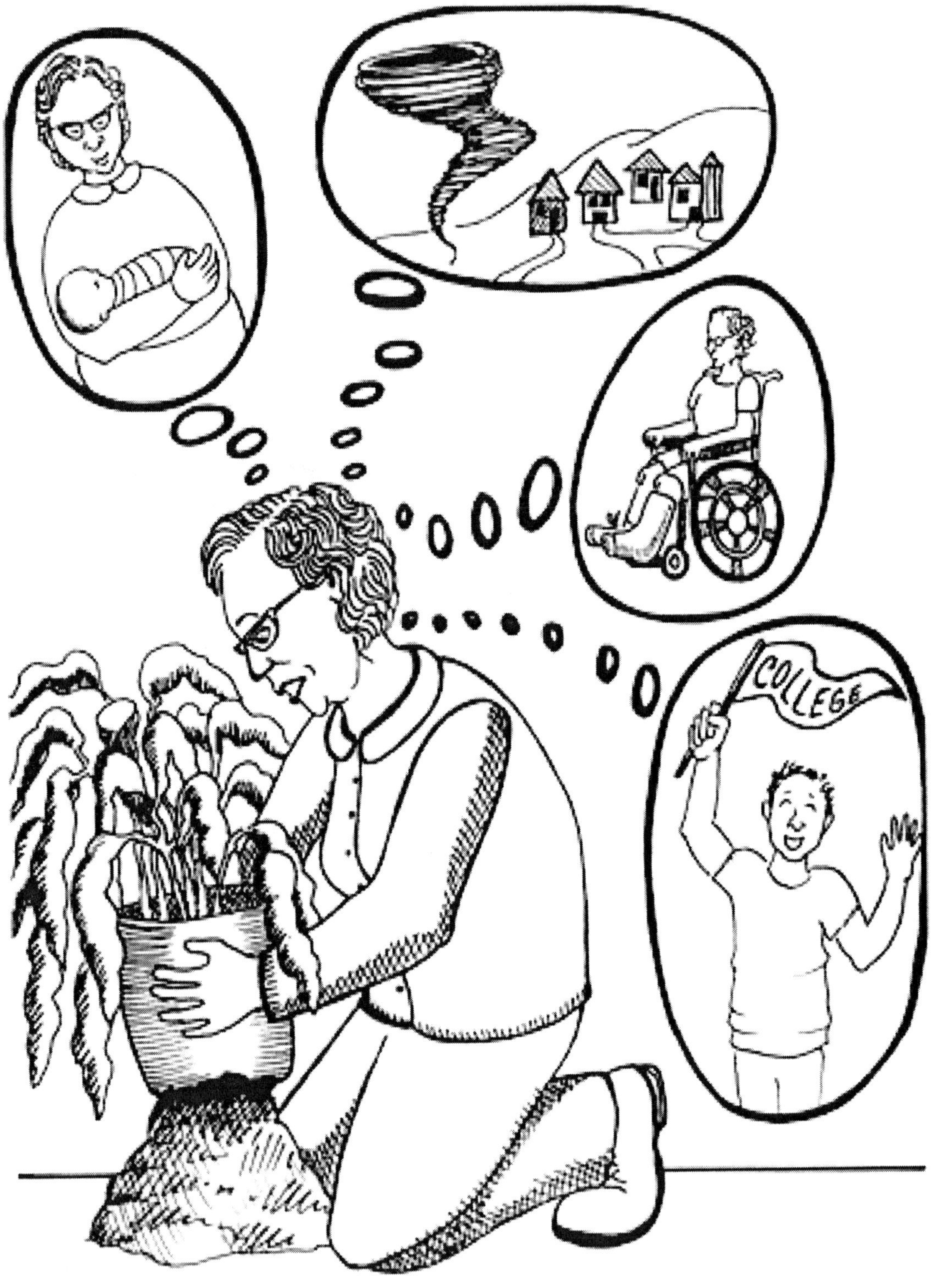
COLLEGE

This was the cycle it followed for the next few years. Years that saw the good and bad stuff of life. The first grandchild was born. A tornado went through the valley but fortunately no one was hurt. Billie fell and broke her leg. The youngest son went off to college and new neighbors came to visit.

All the while that ugly old cactus sat in its coffee can and grew, ever so slowly. During the move onto the porch in the spring when it was six years old, the coffee can was showing its age. It was so rusted and that the images of Mr. Chase and Mr. Sanborn were barely visible.

Billie carefully picked it up to move it to the edge of the porch where it would get more light. That's when the bottom fell out. The soil was all over the floor and the cactus plant lay shattered.

With tears in her eyes she found an old used plastic hanging basket. Tenderly, she sat on the floor and repotted the broken plant. While replanting she saw what looked like the bud for a new stem, but it was different. It was pointed and looked for all the world like a flower bud.

She hung it from the hook in the corner of the porch where she could watch it daily.

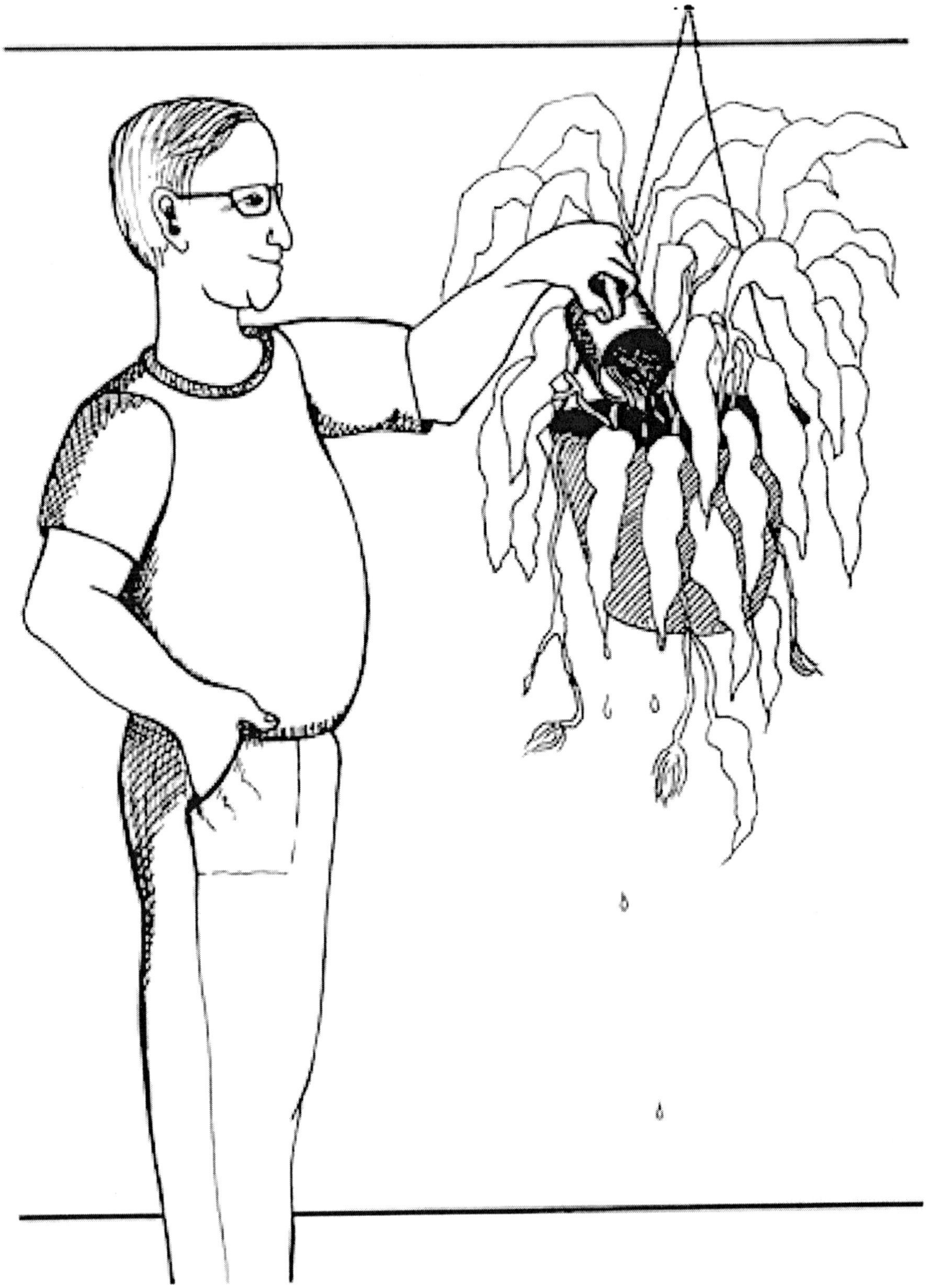

“I think the darn thing’s gonna bloom,” she told Purdy when he came in from the shop. “I didn’t know it got flowers.”

Purdy started slipping out every morning with the remains of a cup of coffee to share with this plant that was finally going to do something. This little dab of coffee was his secret formula, his gift to the cactus about to flower.

They watched the bud grow bigger with each passing day.

“It’s gonna open tomorrow,” Purdy said as they went inside for the evening.

Early the next morning they were both out on the porch. The flower had opened, but now was already beginning to wilt.

“You waited years for a flower that blooms while you’re asleep, lasts one night and is done.” Purdy joked as he poured their coffee.

By noon it was yellowed and spent. That’s all Dottie got to see, a dead flower.

Billie began searching through her garden books and mail order catalogs.

“Here it is!” she shouted to herself. There on the inside back cover of Jung’s seed catalog was a picture of the “Rare and Exotic Night Blooming Cereus, the Queen of the Night.”

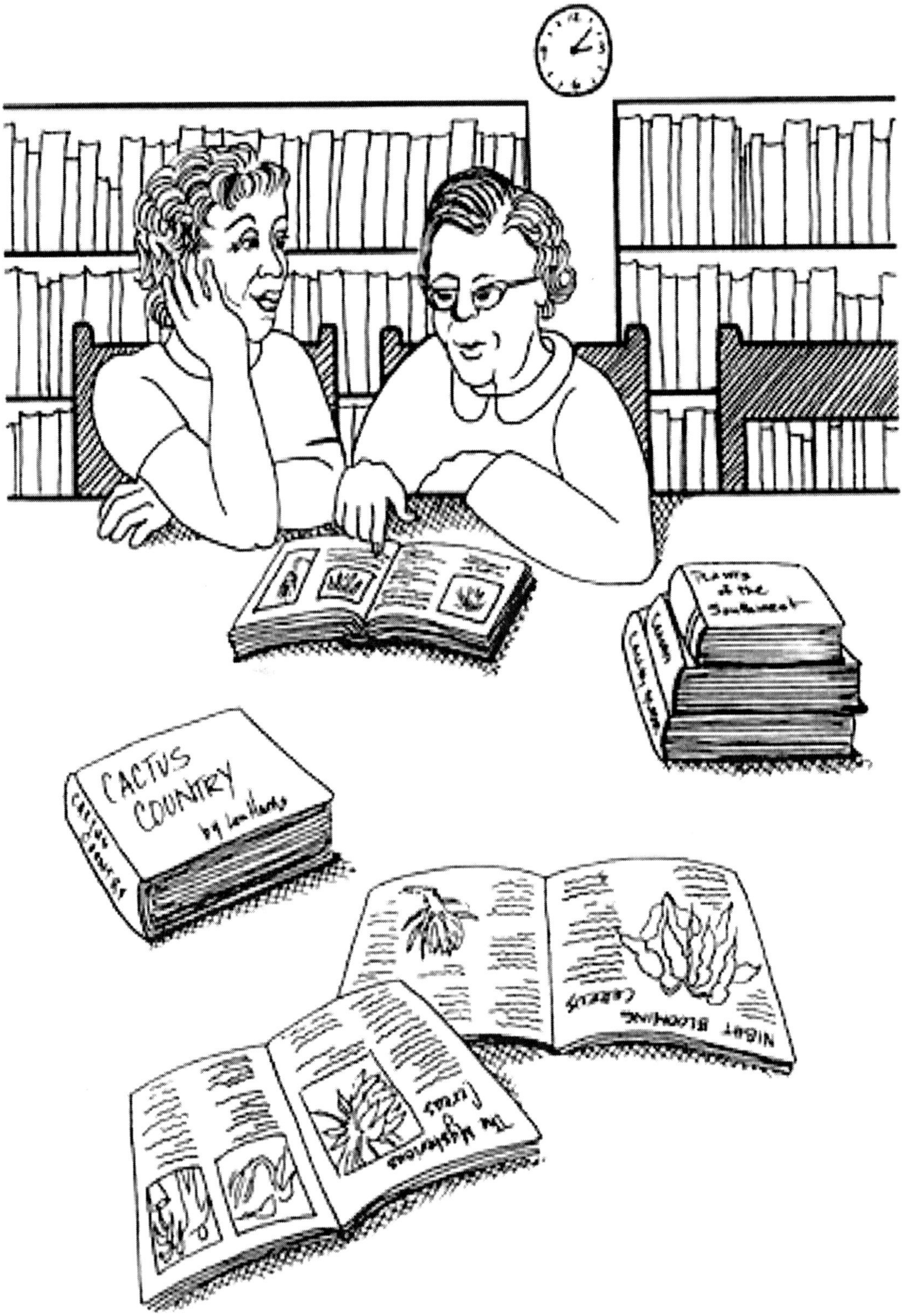
CACTUS COUNTRY
NIGHT BLOOMING CEREUS
The Mysterious Cereus

When Dottie came by, Billie was getting ready to drive to the B. F. Jones Library downtown. Soon these two friends had become experts on the Night Blooming Cereus.

They learned facts that amazed them. It only blooms at night. Each flower lasts only one night. It's pollinated by moths and bats.

"Look at this!" Billy exclaimed, "It says here that it produces fruit that can be eaten."

Dottie leaned over to see the picture Billy was pointing to. "I've gotta see that. Wonder what it tastes like."

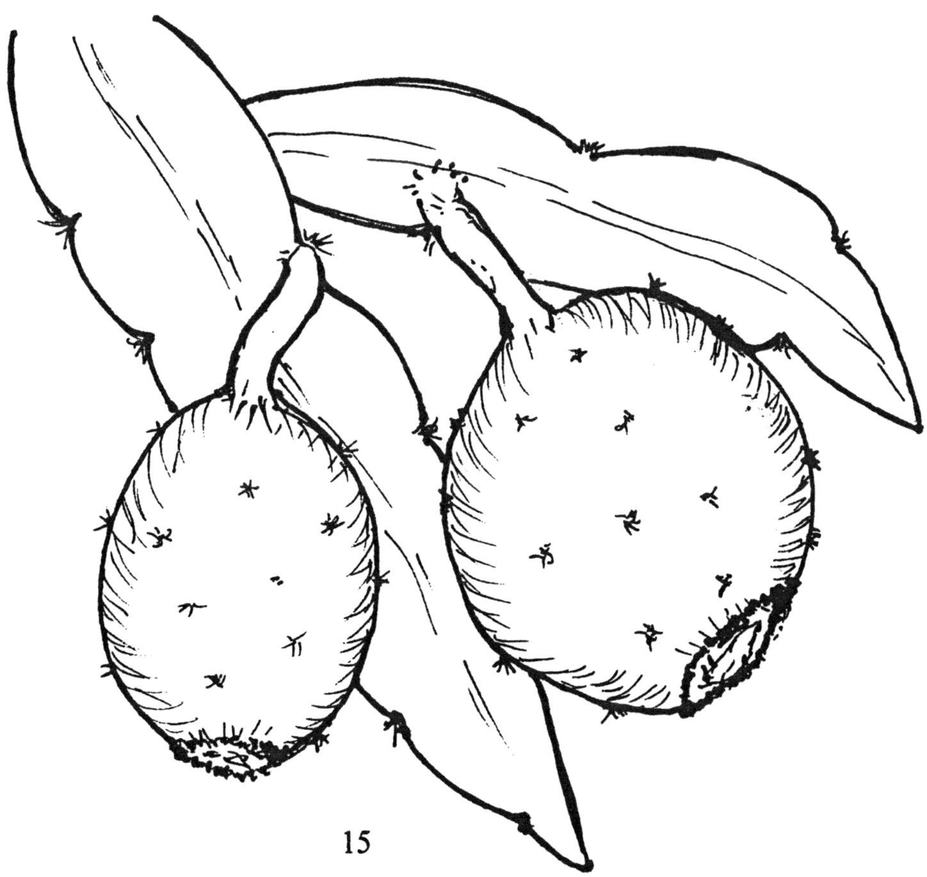

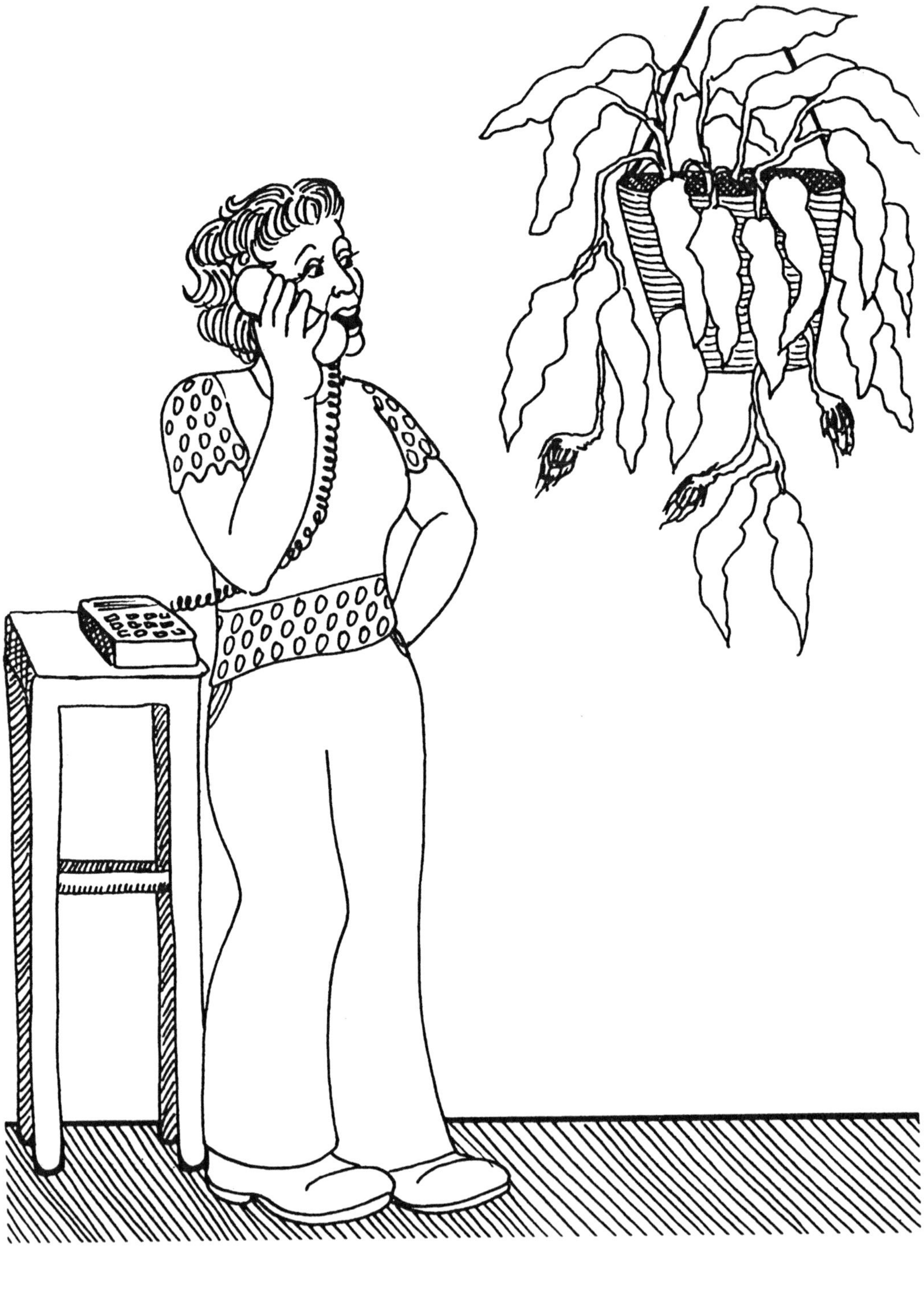

Here it was a year later and this Rare and Exotic Night Blooming Cereus had three buds swelling like little shiny green balloons.

Dottie studied these buds. She had never seen a cactus bloom before, except for a Christmas cactus. By supper time she had called all their friends.

“She’s done it again,” Dottie told them. “Her and that green thumb of hers. Billie’s rare plant is fixin’ to bloom any night now.”

The buds were now almost an inch long, and growing rapidly. Billie was certain that it would open on Saturday evening.

The next afternoon they were planning a party.

Goldie Harwood, now in her eighties, wanted to bring a bouquet from her rose garden and some of her famous apple dumplings.

Hazel and Jim would bring their potato salad, a cheese casserole and their son, Carl. He had Down syndrome but was an artist with a camera. He would record the event.

Petra would bring her summer salad and a wild flower bouquet.

Harriet would bring her home made root beer and a bouquet from her lily garden.

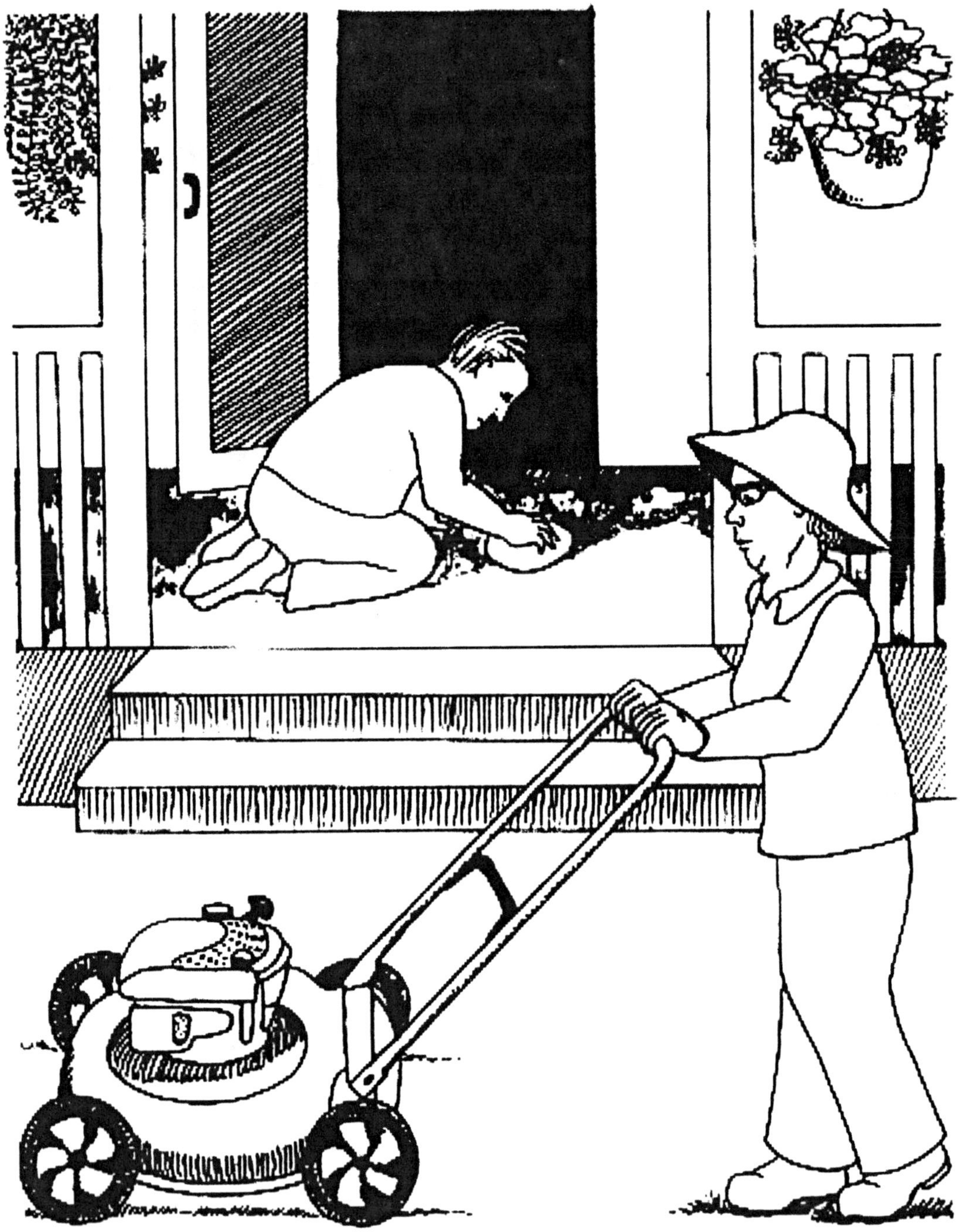

The Dyers promised to bring their popular iced hollyhock tea and a huge bouquet of their most colorful hollyhocks.

Friend after friend wanted to bring something special to make this a most memorable evening.

The old farmhouse had never had this many people visiting at one time. Billie and Purdy scrubbed the floors, mowed the grass, weeded the garden, washed the good dishes and polished the silverware. All the time they were keeping their eyes on the swelling buds.

Friday evening several folks dropped by to check on the buds. Billie was still confident that tomorrow would be the night.

But the weather report was now calling for late afternoon and evening thunder storms. Still, they moved the guest of honor, the Night Blooming Cereus, to the lowest branch in the maple tree.

By noon Saturday there was a steady stream of people coming and going. They were delivering bouquets of flowers, boxes of food, bags of ice and cases of soft drinks.

The neighborhood had never seen anything like this. This was bigger than a family reunion.

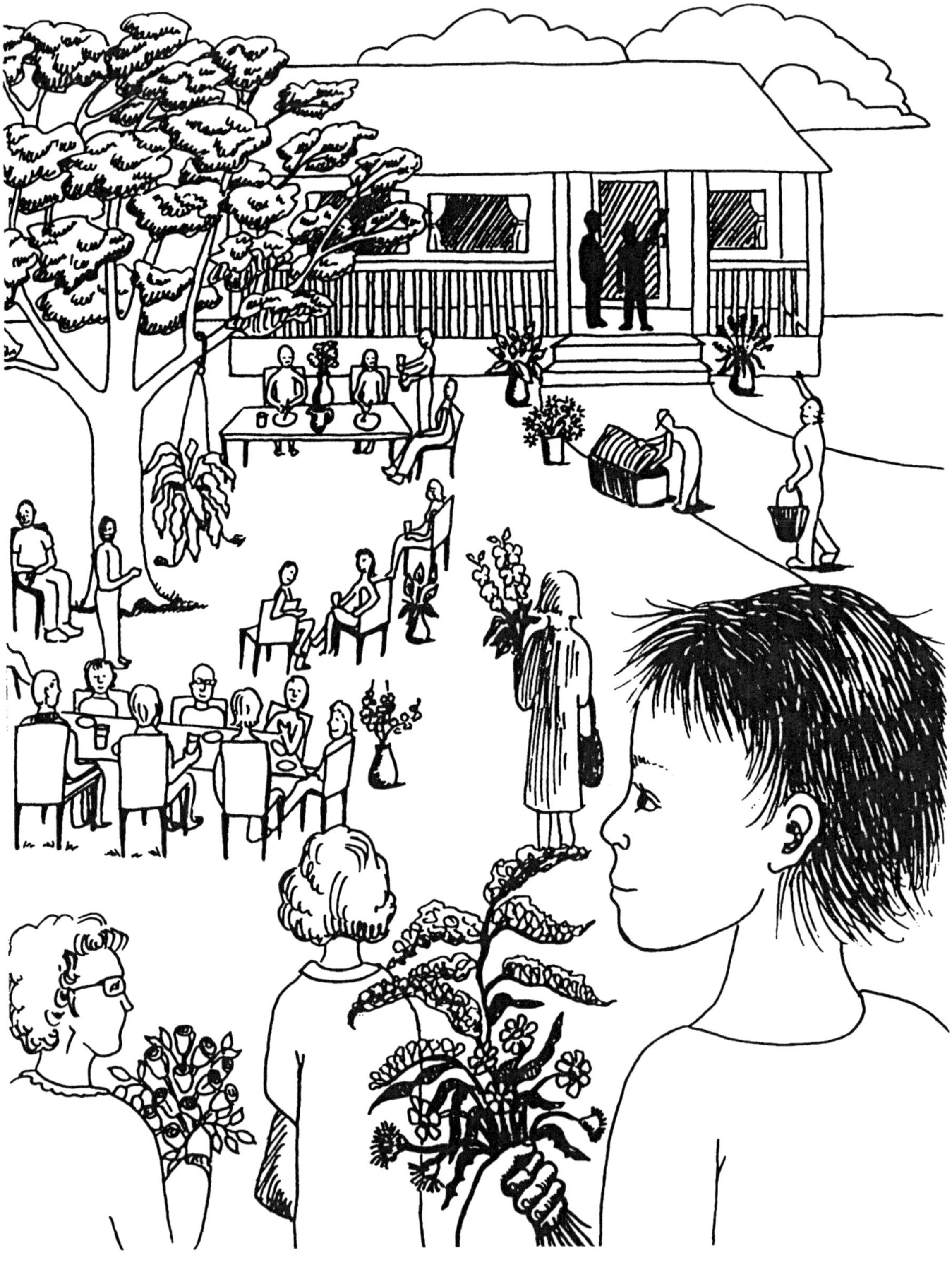

Purdy watched the darkening sky. While they were setting up the tables and chairs under the maple trees the wind began to blow. The Night Blooming Cereus was quickly moved back to the safety of the porch.

Rumbles of thunder could now be heard in the distance. Friends and neighbors continued to arrive. Casseroles, salads, Jello dishes, meatloafs, cakes, pies, and bags of potato chips were stacked on the kitchen table and filled the fridge. Colorful homemade bouquets were sitting everywhere.

Della, a very poor young girl from over the hill, slowly walked into the yard. Some called her 'retarded.' She was shy around all these people.

She often visited Billie, and helped her in the garden. Sometimes she would sit and they would read a book together. Sometimes Billie would sew a new dress for her.

Today Della brought a bouquet of the last of the dandelions and the first of the goldenrods along with a generous helping of bright white daisies. It was all she had to share, but she did it with a shy smile and a whole lot of love.

Billie led Della over to the cactus plant. When Della reached out to touch the waxy bud everyone yelled at her. The tears began to flow.

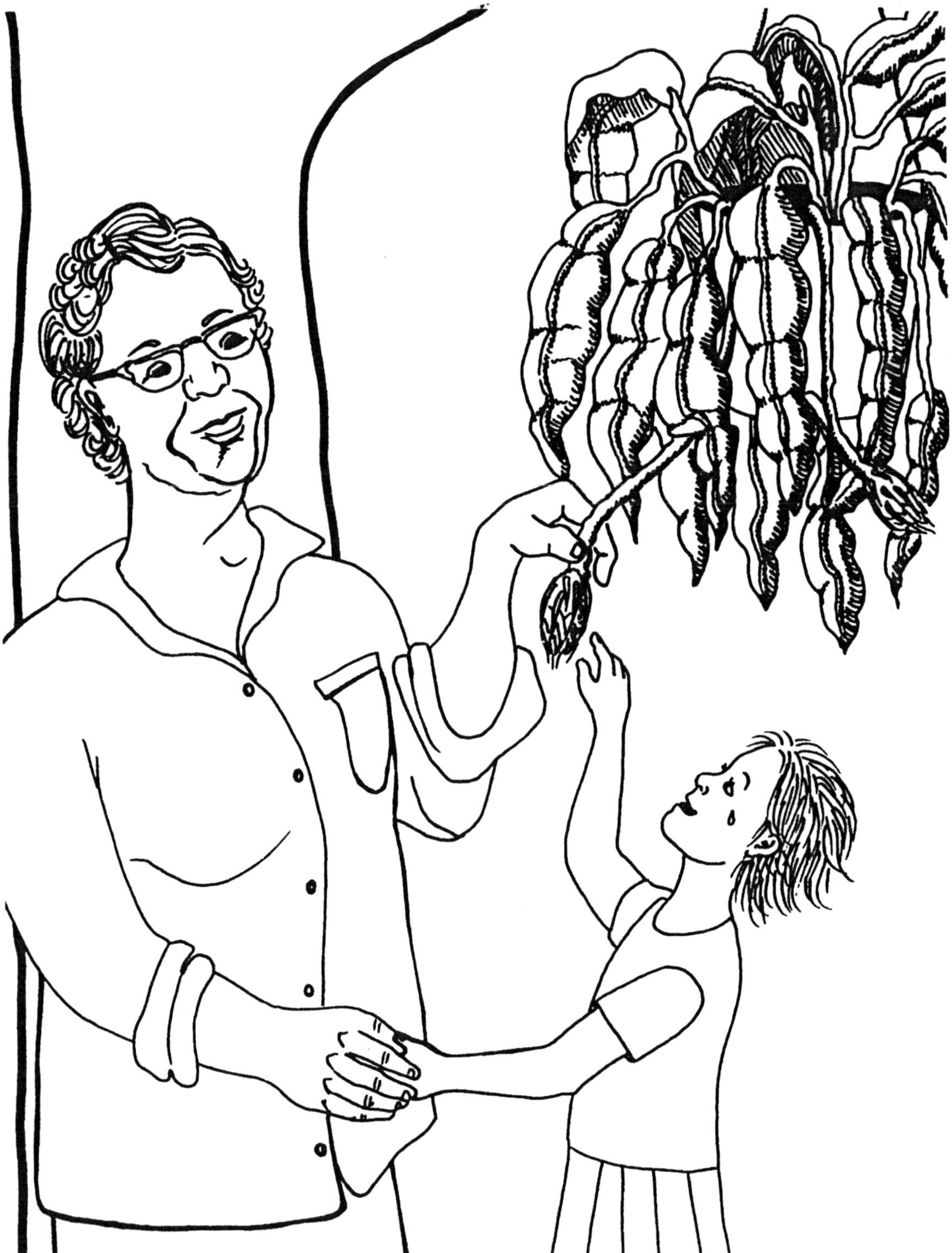

Billie hugged her, wiped away the tears and guided her fingers to gently touch the almost flower. In Billie's mind the little girl was far more precious than the cactus plant's blossom.

Lightning flashed and the thunder shook the ground. The first few drops of rain, big drops, heavy drops, fell on the people and the bouquets that lined the walk and surrounded the porch. Then the wind stopped. The dark clouds moved off to the east and the last of the raindrops disappeared into the grass.

Even while the thunder rumbled its retreat, Billie and Dottie carefully carried the Night Blooming Cereus back to the maple tree. Friends chatted, dined, shared recipes and took turns watching the buds as they continued to expand.

The color had changed from pale green to ivory. Joe Zima began to play a polka on his accordion and several of the people present began dancing in the yard. It was getting dark.

Purdy and Jim lit the candles and placed them on the tables. The bouquets glowed in the candlelight. So did the people. The food was great and the hollyhock iced tea was a big hit.

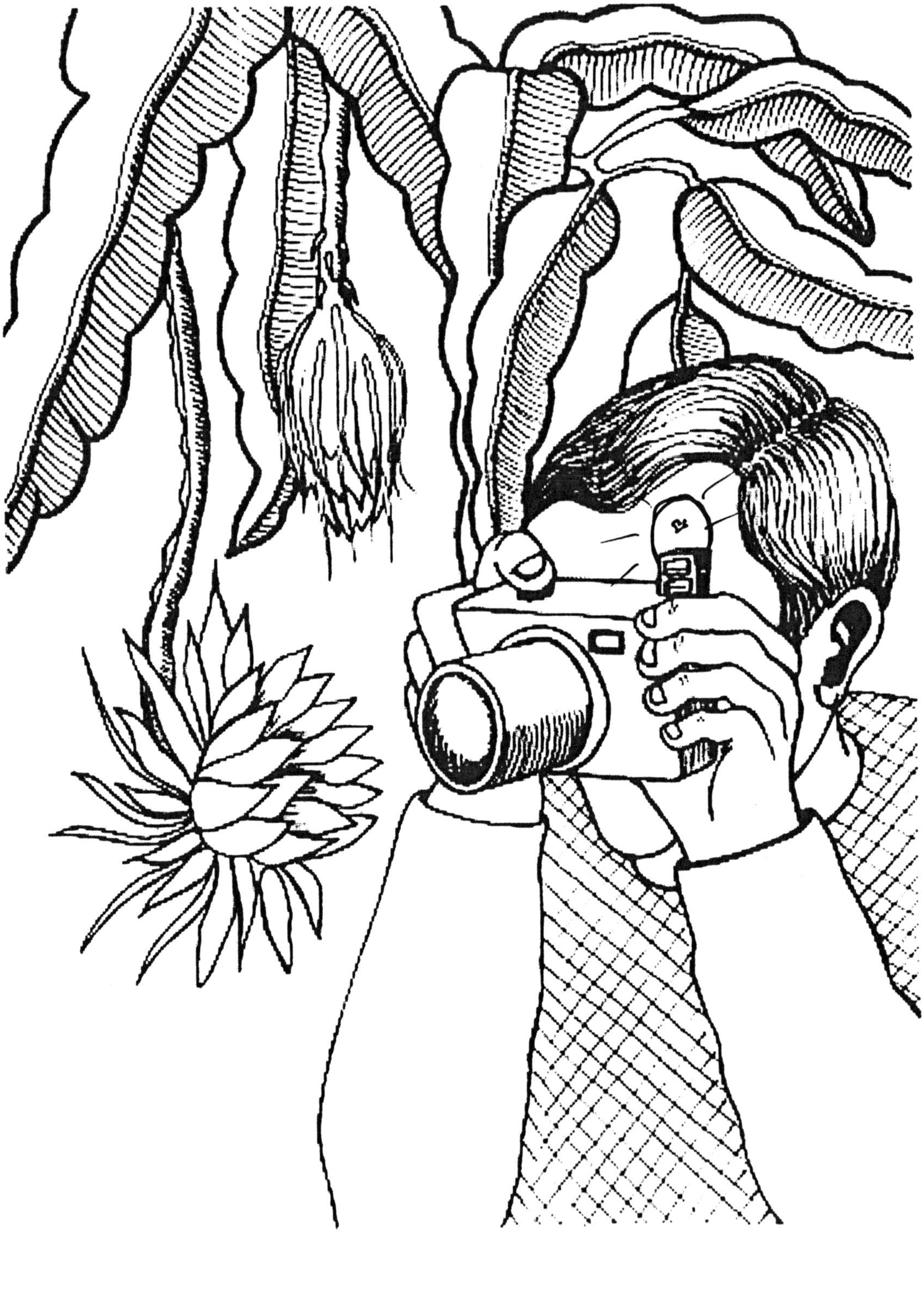

Della had wandered from bouquet to bouquet, smelling the flowers, touching the petals and just being delighted.

Then she looked up at the hanging basket in the maple tree as the first petal burst open. "LOOK! LOOK!" she shouted.

The music stopped. The conversation fell silent and all eyes were on the three buds.

Carl stood at the side, camera ready. As each petal burst from the cluster to claim its freedom, its place in the beauty of the universe, there was the intense light of the flash bulbs. About half of the petals were now open on the first bud.

Everyone was crowded as close as they could get to this magical moment. The first petal burst free on the second bud. Now the challenge was to watch two flowers opening at the same time.

Della tugged at Billie's arm. She bent down and picked up the little girl. Just as Della reached out with one tiny finger the flash bulb exploded and the camera recorded the moment.

The smile on her face was mirrored in Billie's smile.

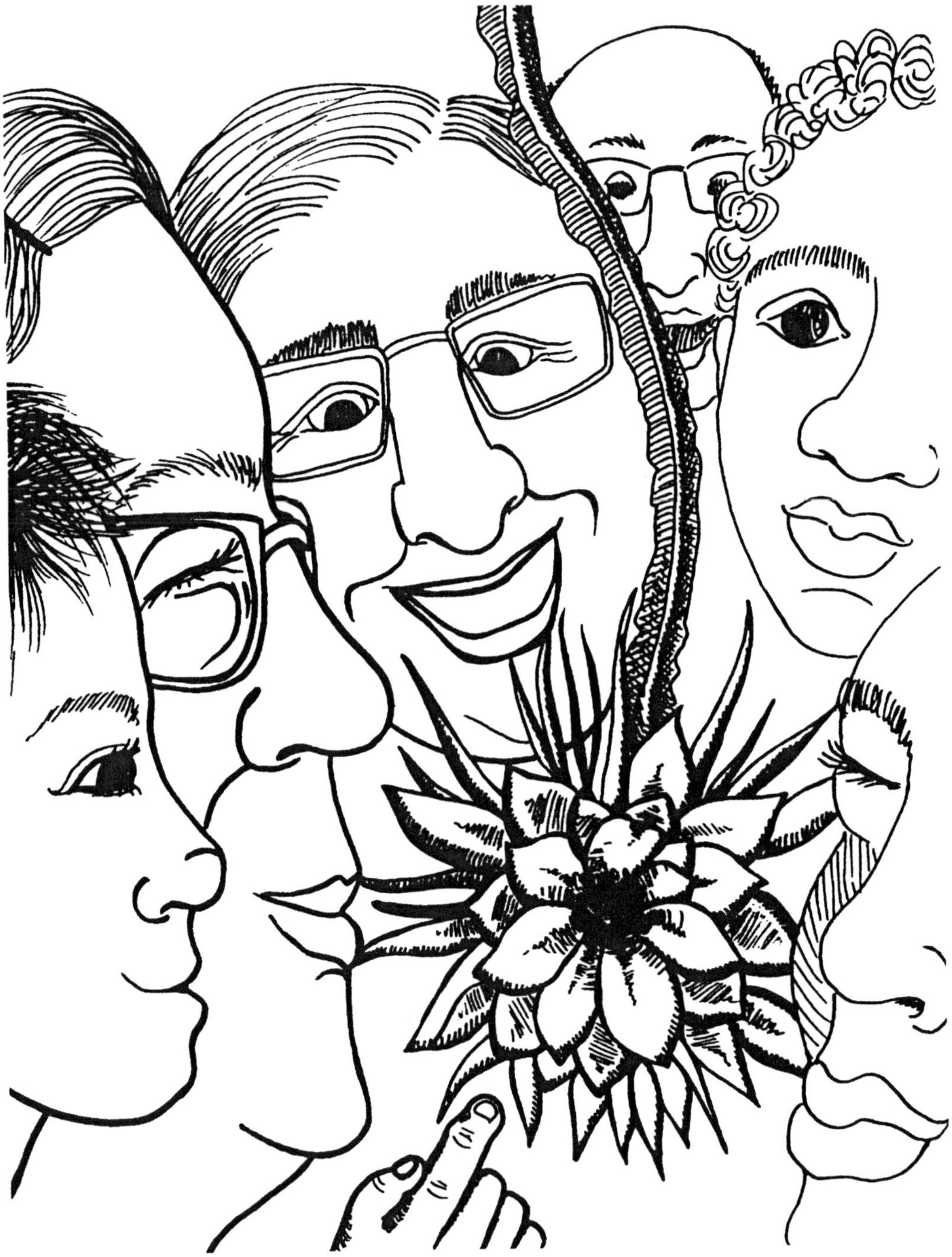

The first bud was finally a flower after about fifteen minutes. The second seemed to open a little quicker.

Billie leaned forward and sniffed the throat of this dynamic glowing white flower. There was a faint, almost lemon scent. Soon everyone was pressing closer to smell and touch this dramatic blossom.

The crowd began to relax and everyone turned back to conversation and food. Billie looked once more at this glowing bouquet of three simple flowers.

There, in the middle of the first flower to open, was a moth. Carl took careful aim. The flash bulb exploded and the moth took flight.

But next week when the film was developed, the photo of the moth on the flower was the second best picture taken that night.

It was the photo of Della touching the first flower that appeared in the local newspaper.

**Author's note:**
**This is based on a true story. You see, Billie was my mother and this story is dedicated to her. Hope you enjoyed this delightful memory. HB**

# Now it's up to you

**❀ Conversation**

We can encourage our family members, fellow residents and staff to share their memories of long awaited events, special flowers or friendly gatherings. There are so many ways to use a story like this as a springboard for discussion. The following are only a few suggestions.

**❀ Activities that can follow the story**

Share stories of an uncommon flower, fruit or vegetable you have grown. Perhaps even begin a quest to find it and grow it again.

❀ Create a "Green Friends" photo album or sketchbook. This can be a joint effort or an individual project. Either way the joy comes in the sharing.

❀ Make an audio recording of this story. Family members, friends or residents of a senior care community can read for each character.

❀ Plan and hold a party for a special plant. It doesn't have to be a night blooming cereus. Perhaps for you it's an orchid, or the first ripe tomato. You can make it a floral seasonal special event. One group actually held a "Dandelion Daze" celebration in honor of this delightful plant. They invited children and played dandelion games, made dandelion flower ice cream and even ate a dandelion salad. They sipped juices through a dandelion stem straw.

**Seniors Illustrated Book Club:**

Some families and senior communities have started a reading club that meets periodically. The stories in this Seniors Illustrated series can be read individually, or aloud to the group. Take the opportunity to discuss the book, share your thoughts and memories, even color the illustrations if you wish. But, most of all enjoy a good story.

# The Great Potato Drop

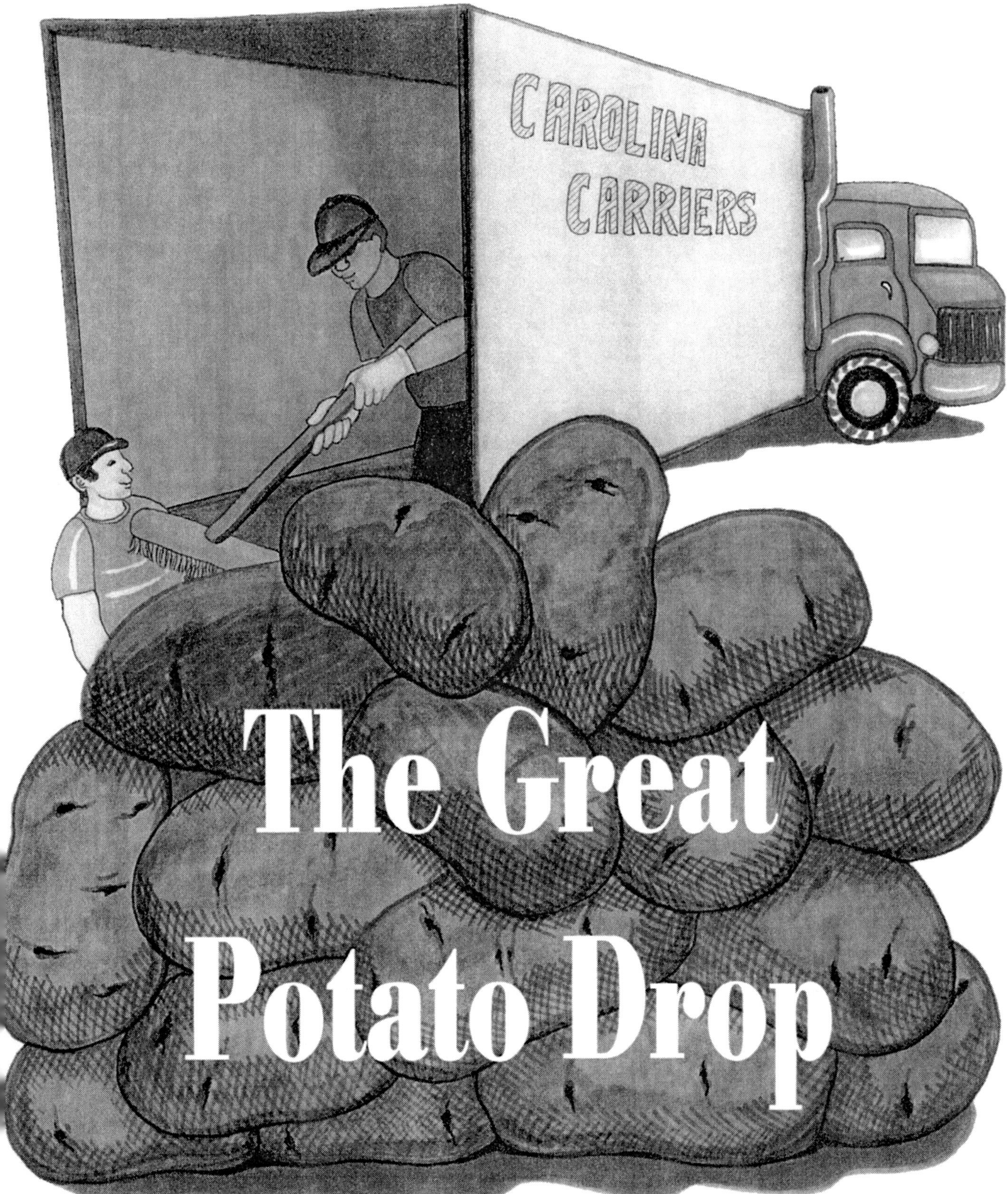

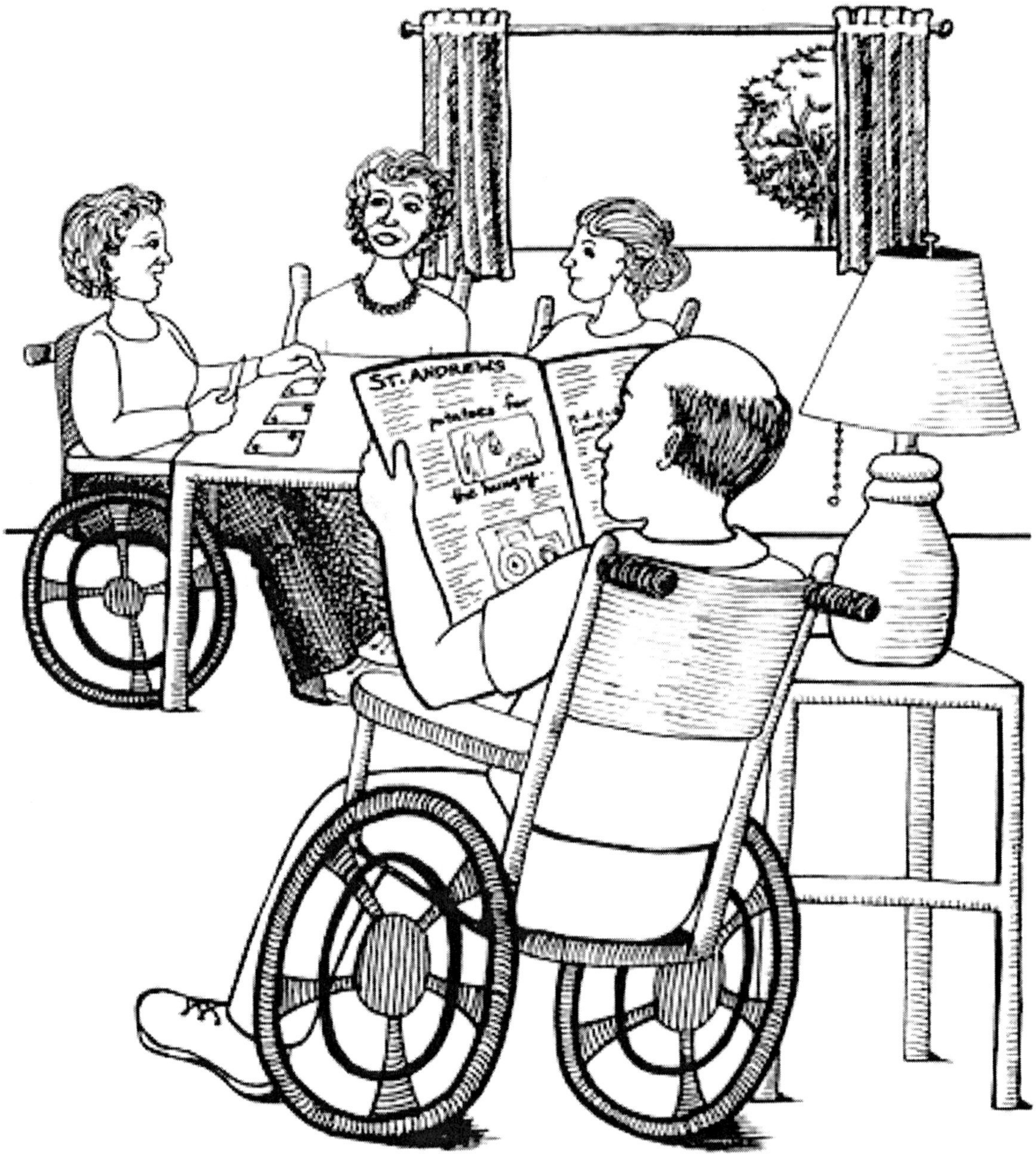
ST. ANDREWS
potatoes for
the hungry

# The Great Potato Drop

The further adventures of the folks at Whispering Winds



It all started when Edgar read the little article in the Sunday paper. "Listen to this," he said. "It's about this organization that does gleaning to provide food for the hungry. With teams of volunteers they harvest the produce left in farmer's fields. They also rescue surplus fruit and potatoes from packing houses."

He paused to see if anyone was listening. Then he continued, "They deliver this healthy food to places where there's a need; soup kitchens, homeless shelters, church food pantries and food banks."

Edgar was a child during the Great Depression. He knew all about hunger, how it destroyed hope and health. Then he read the last paragraph in the article. He waved the paper in the air and shouted to the others in the sitting room.

"Listen to this. These folks, the Society of Saint Andrew. They got truck loads of potatoes in North Carolina that they need to ship to places that can bag them up and distribute them to the hungry."

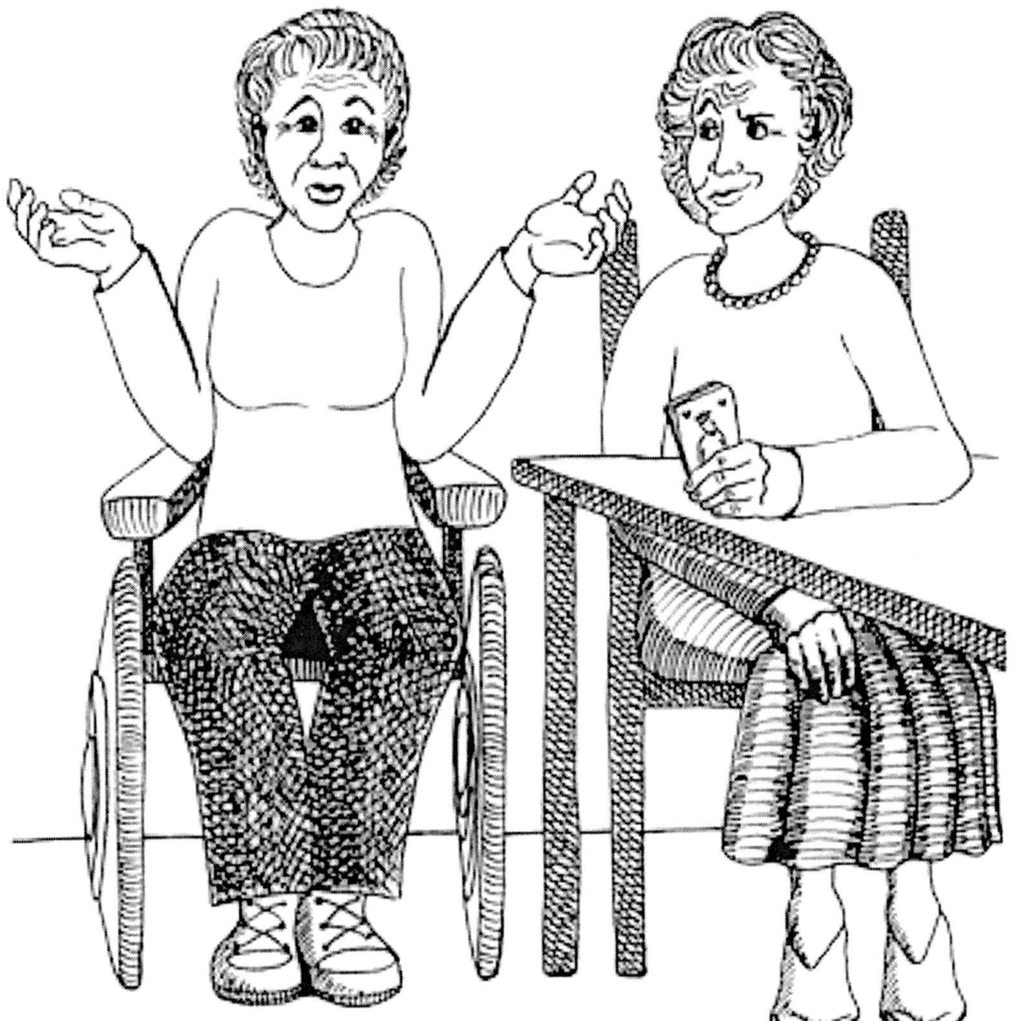

Eunice and Silvia looked at him like he was a stark raving mad lunatic. "So," Silvia said, "What do you want us to do? Do you want us to bag up a truck load of potatoes?"

"Why not?" Edgar responded with a sparkle in his eyes they had never seen before. It was the sparkle of one who has known an empty belly and felt the pain of poverty.

"For one thing," Eunice frowned and grumbled, "We're too old. Another reason is I'm not the only one in this room with arthritis."

Silvia had to point out the obvious, "Look at you. You're in a wheelchair, just like me. How you gonna bag up a truck load of potatoes?"

Edgar smiled at these two women, then, in his soft voice, answered, "One potato at a time. We can invite the whole town to help. If my math is correct, and I did teach math, that works out to about five pounds per person. I think even you could handle that."

As they entered the dining room it was one of those strange twists of fate. The vegetable of the day was, of course, you guessed it, mashed potatoes.

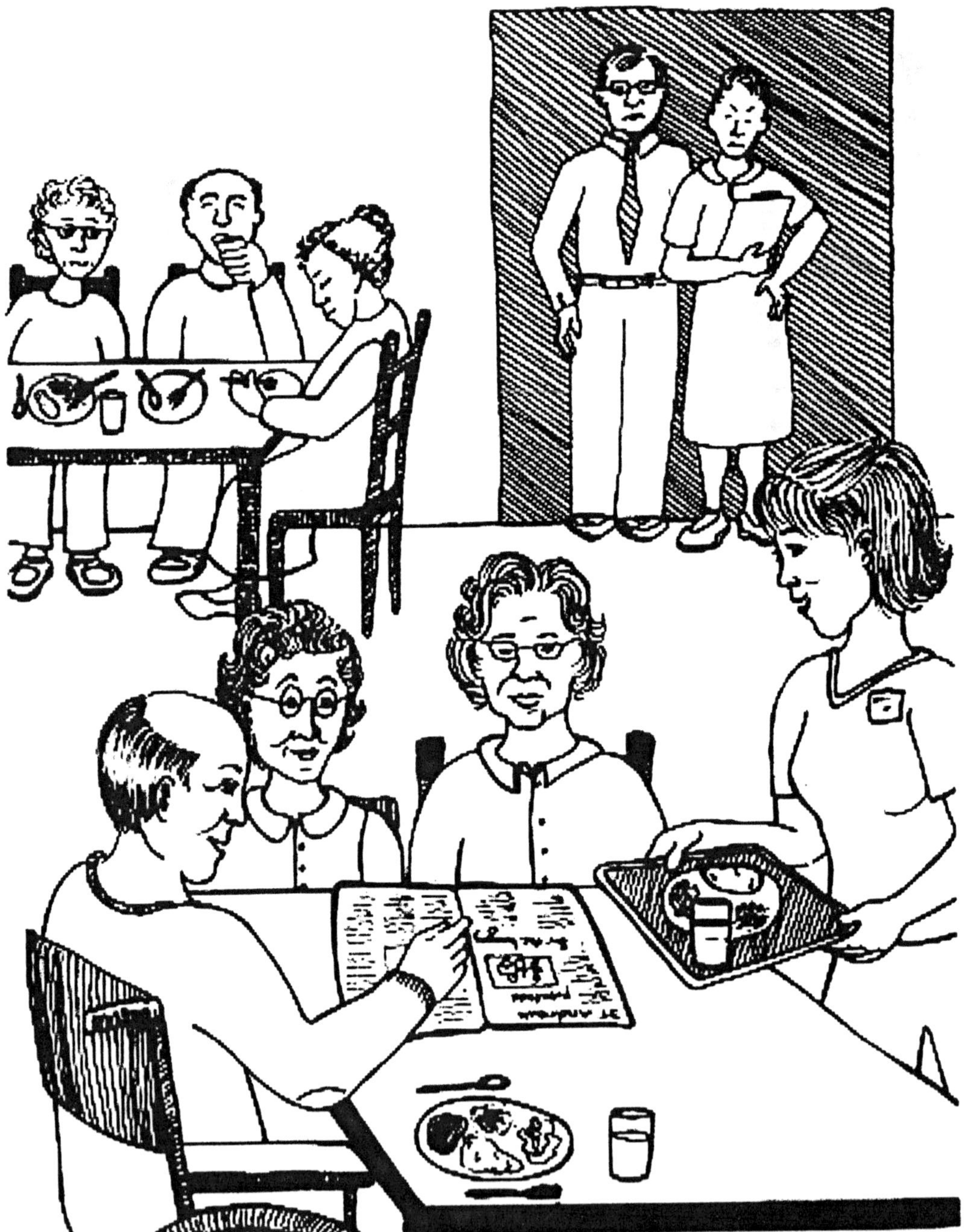

When Edgar mentioned his idea to Nurse Ratchet, she peered over her clipboard. "Hummph, I don't think so," she said and walked away.

Flo and Claire joined Edgar at his table. These two were dangerous when they set their minds to something. Mr. Stewart, the administrator, entered the dining room. They called him Simon Legree because he looked much meaner than he really was. He started worrying the moment he saw Flo and Claire sitting at Edgar's table.

Nurse Ratchet joined him by the door and whispered, "Crazy Edgar wants to bag up a truckload of potatoes." Then she reached for her bottle of antacids.

"Why?" the Whispering Winds' administrator asked. He was convinced that the old math teacher must be completely insane. "What would he do with a truck load of potatoes?"

Joyce was the activity director with the sparkling eyes and a smile that made everyone wonder what she was up to now. She brought her tray to Edgar's table. That's when Nurse Ratchet really began to worry.

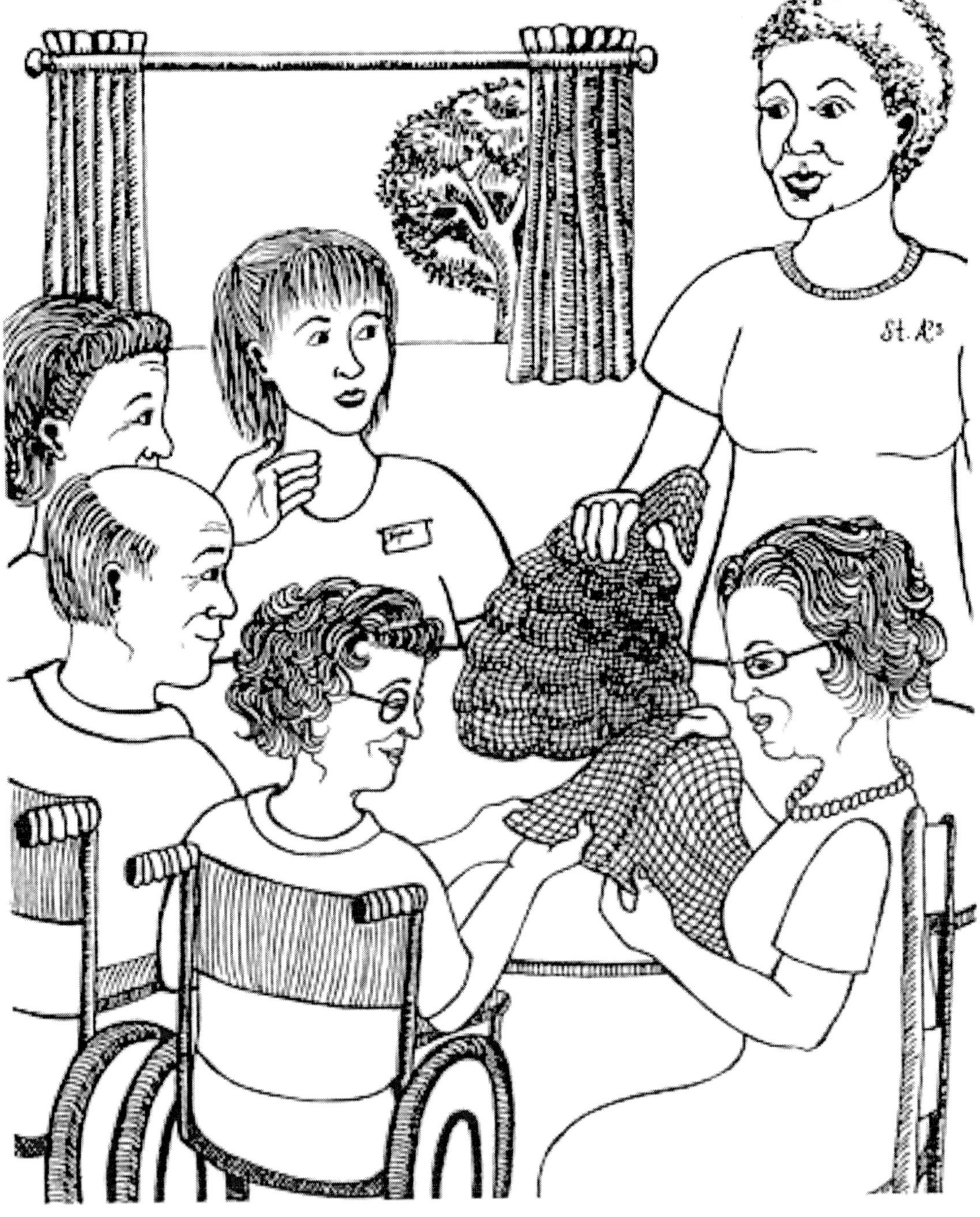

The next few days were filled with phone calls, emails, and visits from a Methodist preacher wearing an orange tee shirt that said "Society of Saint Andrew" in big white letters across the back.

She was carrying a battered briefcase and a 5 lb bag of potatoes. Joyce's assistant led Rev. Bergen into the courtyard where Flo, Claire, Edgar and several other residents were sitting.

Edgar smiled that shy smile of his and motioned her to a seat at the table. She sat the bag of potatoes in front of them. Flo picked it up and studied it closely. "Where do we get the bags?" she asked.

Rev. Bergen, smiled at the group, "Why, you will make them, of course. We'll supply a roll of this mesh material," she said, "and you will cut it up and stitch the bottom. We will need about 9,000 bags for a load of potatoes."

Edgar leaned forward in his wheelchair, "I think we can get the whole town involved in this project. I have already called the high school, and the scouts are eager to help out."

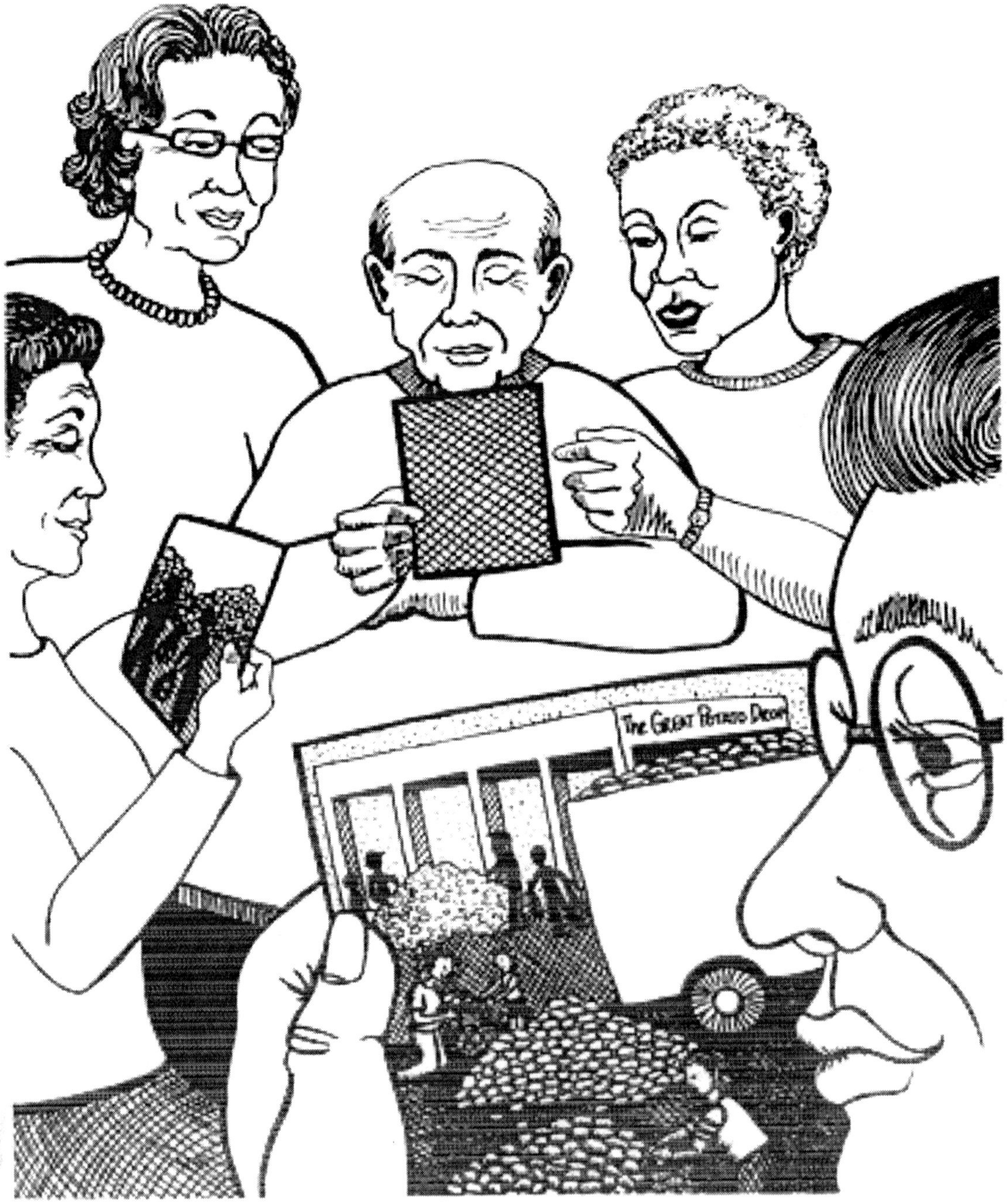
The Great Potato Drop

"I have been calling the churches, and it looks like all the Sunday school classes and the youth groups are on board," Claire added.

"The Haitian farm workers also want to help, and we called the garden clubs," Flo smiled, as she fingered the mesh stitching that secured the bottom of the bag, "and my daughter, she's a special ed teacher, wants to get her students involved too."

"How does this work?" Edgar asked.

The preacher opened a large envelope and removed a series of 8 x 10 photos. The first showed a large truck filled to overflowing with potatoes. The next showed a truck dumping all those potatoes onto the pavement of a school parking lot. Another showed children filling bags, tying them shut and piling them on wooden pallets.

"We will pay for the delivery costs and contact local soup kitchens, food pantries, and food banks that can distribute them. We do ask you to help us recruit teams to help with the bagging and clean up."

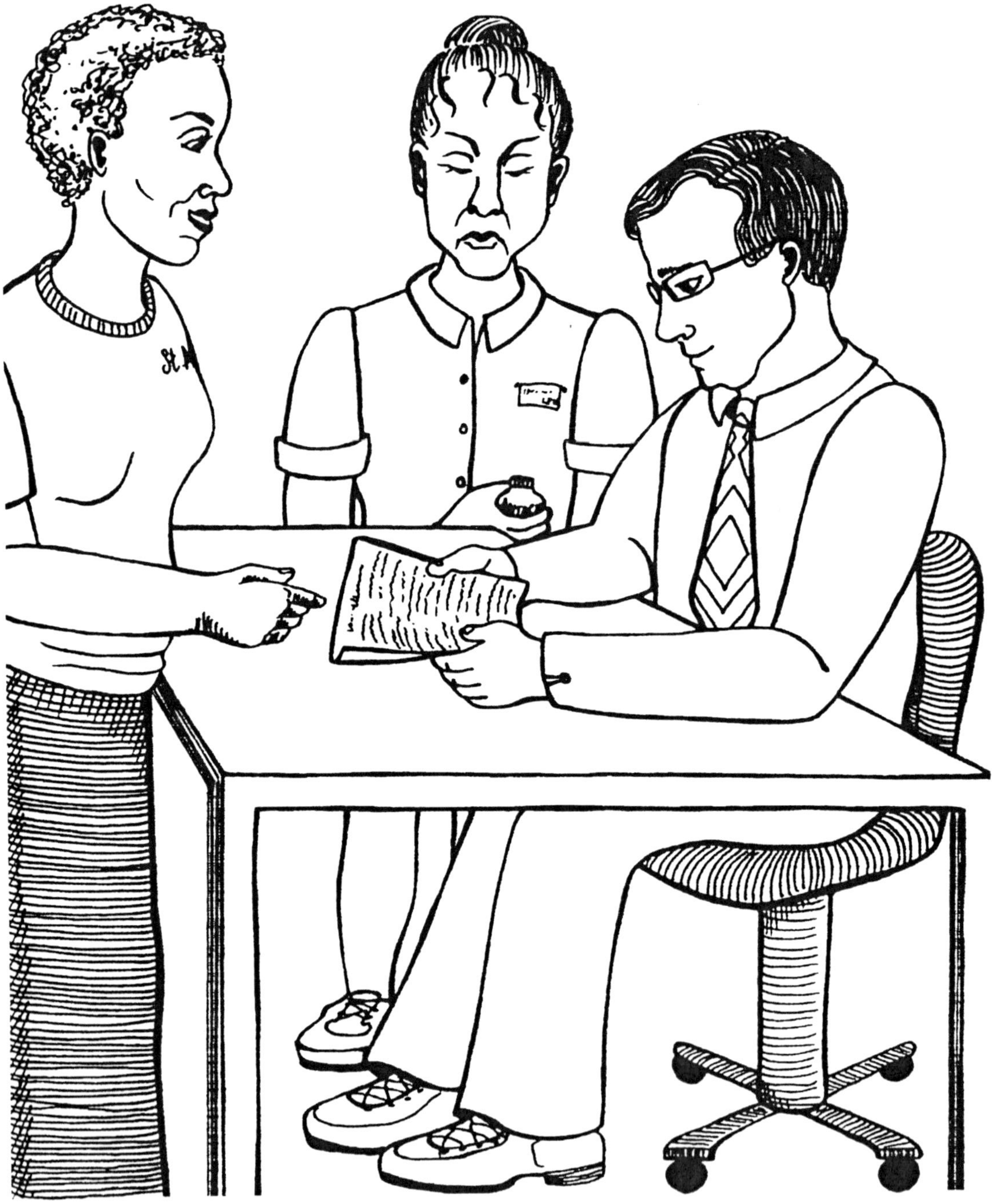

Rev. Bergen leaned back and studied the elders at the table. "We've never done this at a nursing home before. We're going to have to depend on you all to show us how."

She was looking at Edgar, Flo and Claire, not Joyce and Polly.

Simon Legree was concerned about health issues, the chances of injury or fainting in the summer heat. Lawsuits and bad publicity were his greatest fears.

Still the idea intrigued him. He wanted to know more about this crazy idea. Nurse Ratchet joined him with her ever-present bottle of antacids and scowl.

Later Rev. Bergen stopped by Simon Legree's office and handed him a packet of paperwork that needed to be signed before they could begin planning for this "Great Potato Drop."

In the next week Edgar, Flo and Claire spread the word to all the residents of Whispering Winds.

Claire created a poster on the computer and printed out enough to post them on every door.

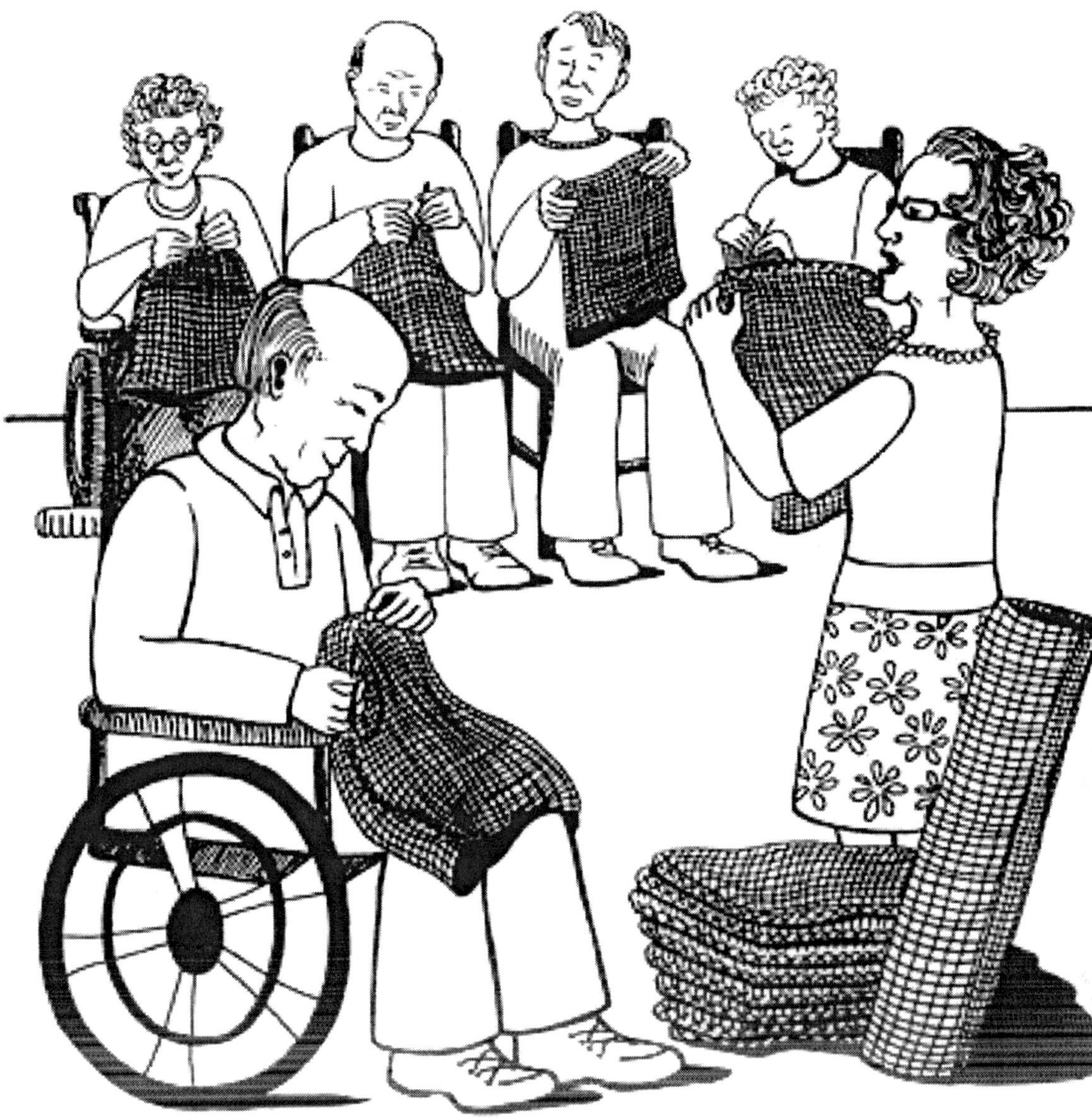

Flo and Joyce drew up a letter to send out to every business and organization they could think of in town, and in neighboring towns.

Two weeks later the rolls of mesh arrived. The next afternoon they had an assembly line set up. Flo kept telling everyone, "Stitching the bottom of the bag is just like working with plastic canvas."

The businesses were calling Joyce to offer cold drinks, tents, donuts, fans, and employees to help on the big day.

An array of musicians, country singers, a rock band and a Scottish piper all offered their services to entertain the "bag ladies."

In less than two weeks all 9,000 of the bags were stitched and ready. Volunteer baggers were eager for word that the truck was on its way, and the local newspaper had already run the first article on this event.

Rev. Bergen had organized a convoy of trucks to haul the potatoes to soup kitchens, food pantries and homeless shelters. Everyone was waiting impatiently for the truck to arrive.

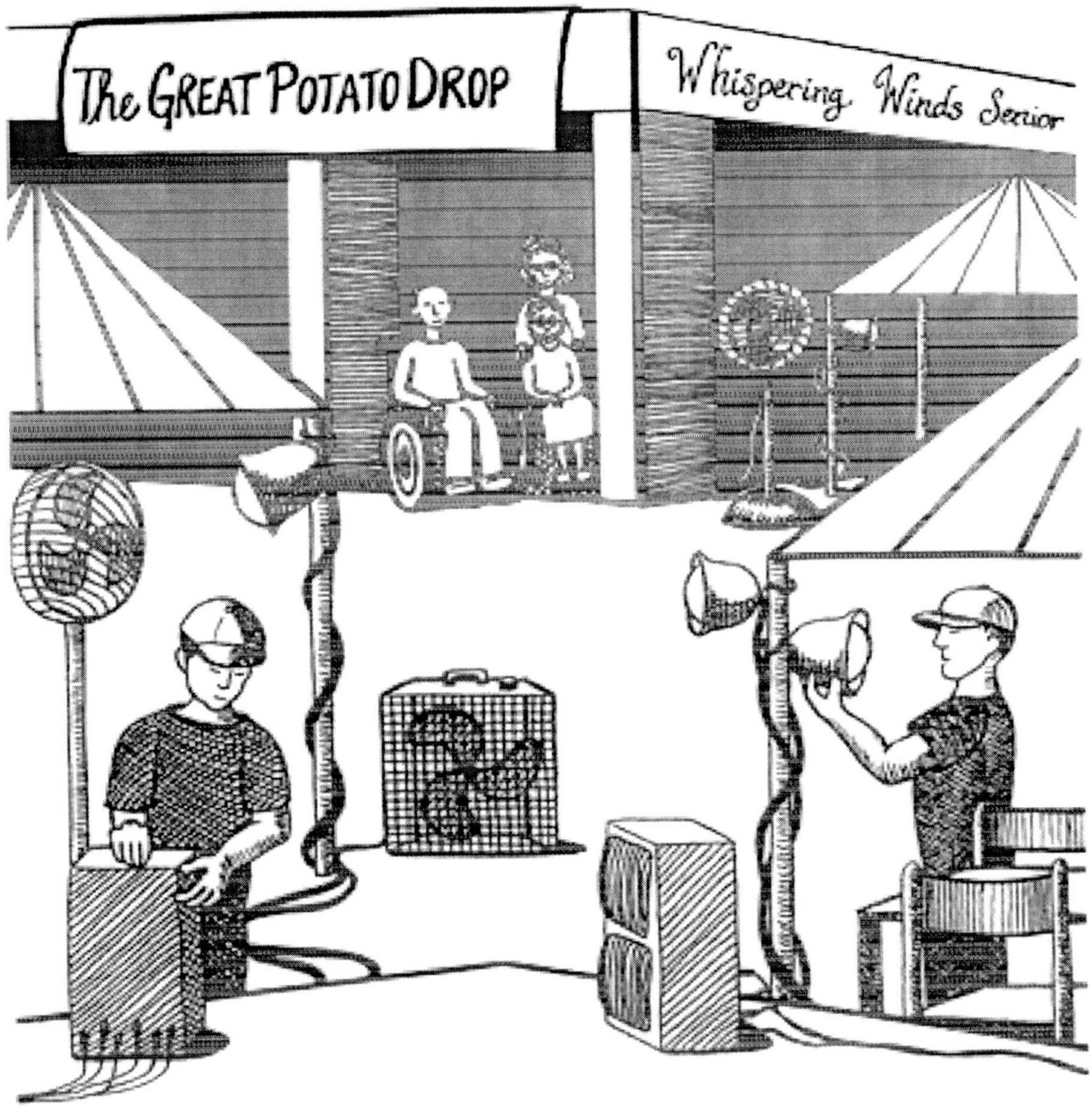
The GREAT POTATO DROP
Whispering Winds Senior

For two more weeks everyone waited. Edgar, Flo and Claire were getting worried. In fact, they were downright antsy.

Finally Rev. Bergen called. The truck had left North Carolina at 6:00 AM that morning with 45,236 pounds of potatoes. It was estimated that it would arrive in two days.

Tents were set up, extension cords were run for the fans and lights in case this project ran into the late evening. The sound equipment was set on the makeshift stage at the entrance to Whispering Winds.

It was amazing how fast it all came together. That evening, at the dinner table, Edgar had a look of apprehension on his face.

“What’s the matter?” Claire asked as she sat her tray on the table.

“What if it doesn’t work?” he said. “What if these potatoes are all rotten?” What if nobody shows up to help?” He looked really worried.

Claire laughed, “Then, I suppose, we are all gonna eat a heap of potatoes for the next few weeks.”

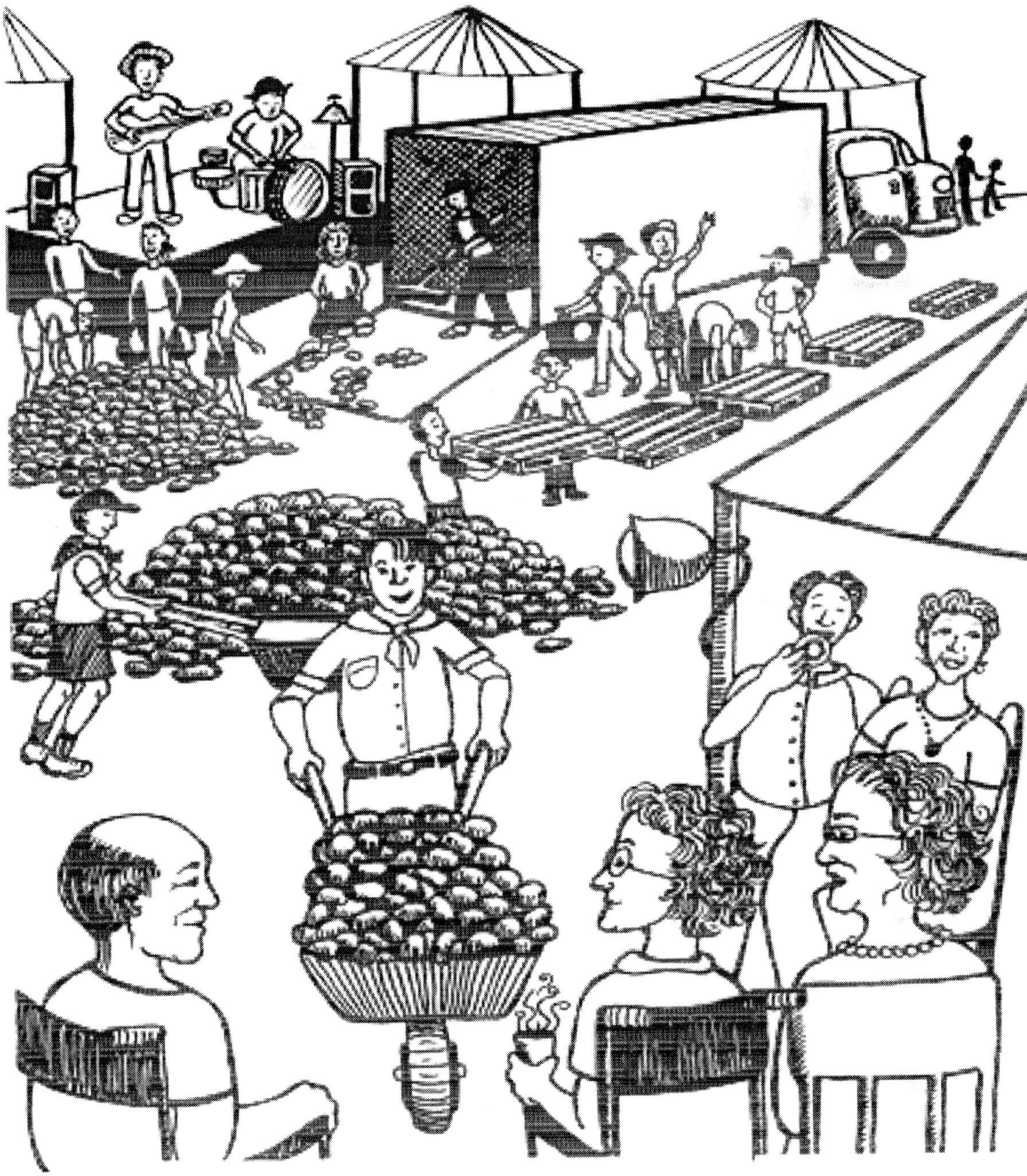

But they didn't have any reason to worry. When the huge truck arrived in the parking lot at 6:15 the next morning, there were over two hundred people already waiting.

By the time the truck had dumped this load in the empty lot, another hundred had joined them.

As the last of the potatoes rumbled and rolled out of the huge truck, the first of the singers began playing his guitar and singing the John Denver song "I Want to Live."

Before the truck pulled back onto the highway, the boy scouts had already begun delivering wheelbarrow loads of the potatoes to the tables under the first tent.

Seated there were over thirty of the Whispering Winds residents, waiting with coffee cups and donuts in hand. Piles of mesh bags sat beside them.

Meanwhile, some of those gathered in the parking lot were laying out the pallets. Others were forming lines to bag potatoes, then hand them off to the stackers at the pallets and loading areas. Everyone was eager to get started.

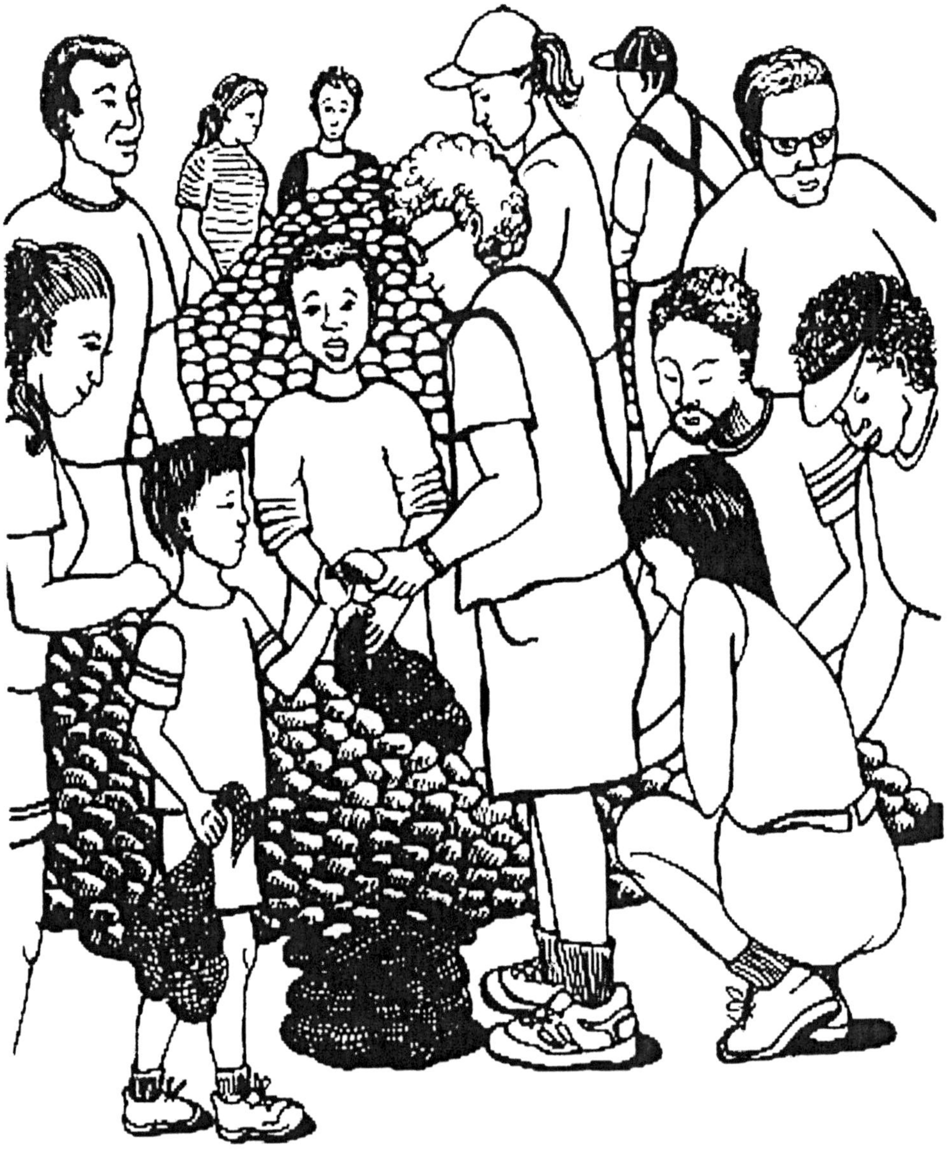

People of every age, from four or five to over ninety were a part of the GREAT POTATO DROP. There were people in wheelchairs, veterans with missing limbs, a group from the school for the blind, several garden clubs and groups of city workers on these lines.

A group from the homeless shelter worked alongside the employees of the local bank. Retirees and first graders worked together.

It was a delightful rainbow of colors as people of all races and nationalities were working, talking and laughing with each other. Conversations were carried on in Greek, Ukrainian, Spanish, Creole, Vietnamese, Chinese, Indian and English.

Trucks of every sort and size were lined up to be loaded. The music became louder as the morning progressed. Donuts gave way to salads, iced tea and baskets of fresh fruit.

By 1:00 PM all the potatoes were bagged. What hadn't already been delivered was waiting on the pallets. Almost four hundred people were sweating in the midday sun. A local radio personality had replaced the live music. Not because the musicians were tired.

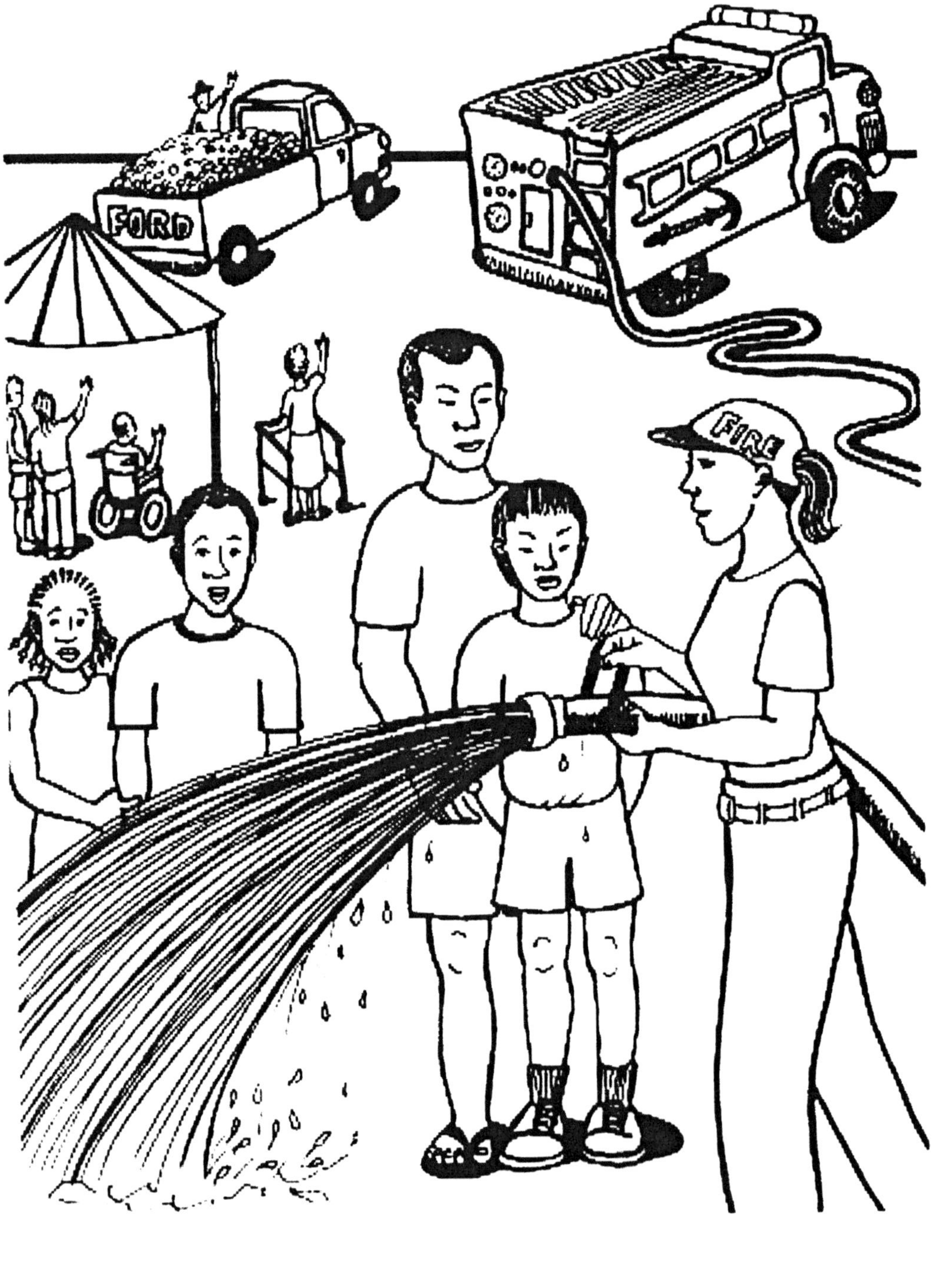
FORD
FIRE

No, they wanted to do their share of the 'potato baggin'.

About a pick up truck load of damaged and spoiled potatoes was left in the middle of the lot and a farmer was on his way to collect these for his hogs. The fire truck was waiting for this farmer's arrival so that they could hose down the parking lot.

It was front page news in the local newspaper, with full color photos of every one smiling, singing, and dancing around the piles of potatoes. A community had come together, not in crisis, not to confront a disaster, but to simply help each other.

The TV Action News team was on the scene from the truck's arrival until the last bag had been picked up. The Great Potato Drop was the featured story with all the details on the News at 10.

Simon Legree, Mr. Stewart, was interviewed. When the TV reporter began praising his great idea of organizing "The Great Potato Drop" at Whispering Winds, Mr. Stewart led the reporter to the tent.

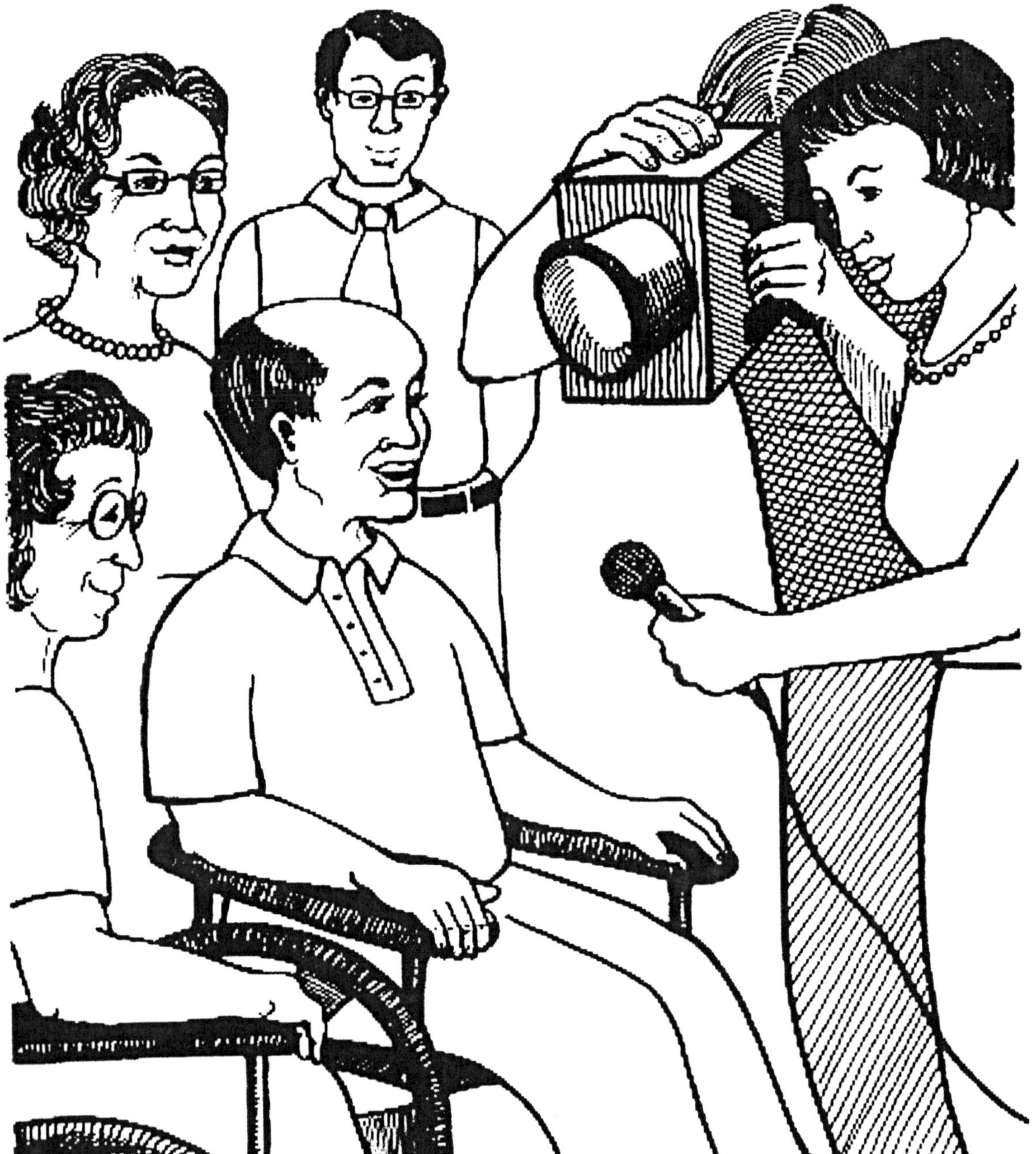

“Here are the real heroes,” he said patting Edgar, Flo and Claire on the shoulder. “It was their idea, and they made it work.”

“Look around you,” he continued, “There are heroes of every size, age and description here.”

During the interview Edgar smiled and stated, “Good news does happen, but only when we make it happen.”

Edgar, Flo, Claire and over fifty fellow residents of Whispering Winds had bagged over 1,000 five pound bags themselves.

Because they had the courage to do something good, over twenty tons of potatoes were now on the way to feed the hungry, homeless and a little less hopeless. If a small group of senior citizens, residents of a nursing home, hadn’t seized the initiative, over twenty tons of nutritious food would have ended up in a landfill.

**This story is based on a true event that occurred in Central Florida several years ago. But it can happen anywhere that there are heroes willing to make it a reality.**

The residents of Whispering Winds were so happy at the day's outcome, they made this poster to send to all groups who had participated:

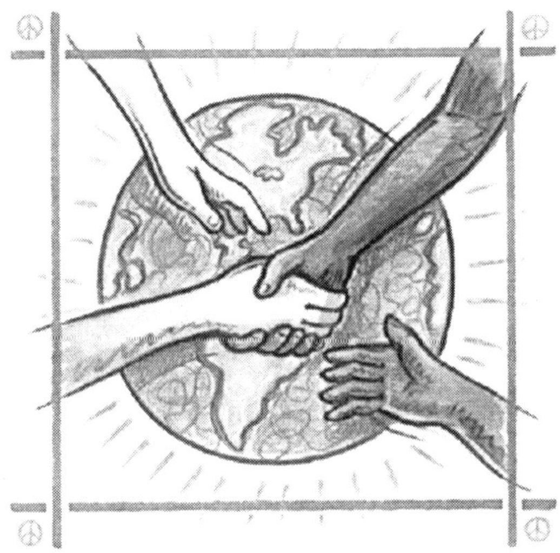

**Thanks for Your Helping Hands**

**caring, loving hands;**
**reaching, sharing hands;**
**hands with calluses worn;**
**hands just newly born;**
**elegant, arthritic, old;**
**youthful, hopeful, bold;**
**hands brown and black and white**
**worked together in God's sight;**
**hands in prayer, folded tight,**
**then open wide instead,**
**providing daily bread.**

The poem is ©1998 by Tomi Jill Folk.

## Now it's up to you:

One of the Green Thumb Clubs in a senior community was left on their own one afternoon when the activity director was caught in traffic. They were meeting in the room beside the kitchen and in a matter of minutes their creative minds were on a rampage. It all started when a bag of potatoes was spotted sitting in the doorway. Soon potatoes were spread across the table. Conversation was spontaneous and contagious. First they compiled a list of ways to eat potatoes and took a vote to see which was the most popular. This is a fun project for any group to do.

Maria Lucero changed the discussion when she began telling a story about how her grandmother would place slices of potato on her forehead if she had a headache or a fever. "This would work most of the time," she explained. Soon others were sharing their potato stories, like the way Colleen's Irish uncle would remove warts with a potato. And there were many others.

Next one of the club members left the room and returned minutes later with a handful of table knives and spoons. She showed them a project they had done when she was a student in a little one room school in Ohio. They then set to work cutting their potatoes in half. Next, on the clean flat surface they began to carve images of flowers, shapes or geometric patterns. Then they "borrowed" some paint and dipped their "potato stampers" in the paint, then onto some plain white muslin that had been reserved for a craft project. For some it was a mess, for others it was art, but for everyone, it was fun.

## Just a couple thoughts:

Do you remember the elementary school science experiment where you made a "potato battery" to power a small clock or radio? How did that work anyway?

Have you ever made a 'Patriotic Potato Salad? It's both fun and easy. You start with red skin potatoes, white potatoes and blue potatoes. You can add any other vegetables you have on hand.

Have you ever grown or eaten blue potatoes? Try it.

# Mashed Potatoes

a little just for fun trivia quiz

The potato is the most popular vegetable in America, and the fourth most popular food in the world after wheat, rice and corn. Let's see how well you know this versatile vegetable.

1. Potatoes are sometimes called SPUDS
a) in honor of the famous "people's interviewer, Spuds Terkel.
b) from a South America Indian word that means "tastes good."
c) a play on a medical term for "sleeping with your eyes open."
d) an Irish term for a type of shovel used to dig potatoes

2. When was Mr. Potato Head born?
a) 1929
b) 1888
c) 1952
d) 2020

3. The potato is related to
a) the sweet potato
b) onions
c) turnips
d) tomatoes

4. Potatoes originated in
a) South America
b) Spain
c) Ireland
d) Africa

5. Potatoes have been used to cure a number of illnesses, diseases and conditions. Such as
a) warts
b) headache
c) rheumatism
d) toothache

6. The potato was poorly received when introduced to France because it was thought to cause
a) Leprosy
b) Sterility
c) blindness
d) left-handedness

7. Americans eat an average of
a) 1 lb of potatoes a week
b) 1 potato a day
c) 1 ton a year
d) 1 serving of McDonald's French Fries a week

8. French fries were first served at the White House by
a) Benjamin Franklin
b) Teddy Roosevelt
c) George W. Bush
d) Thomas Jefferson

9. The Potato Capital of South Dakota is the town of Clark. This town is home to
a) the International Potato Museum
b) the largest potato ever grown
c) the world famous Mashed Potato Wrestling Contest
d) the Russet Family Potato Farm

10. Someone who spends all his or her time sitting and watching the TV is commonly called
a) a cold potato
b) a couch potato
c) a fat potato
d) a potato brain

11. Potatoes produce lavender-blue star shaped flowers. These blossoms became a fashion statement when who wore them in her hair?
a) Queen Elizabeth II
b) Jackie Kennedy
c) Mary Todd Lincoln
d) Marie Antoinette

12. Which vice president misspelled p-o-t-a-t-o by adding a 'e' at the end?
a) Al Gore
b) Dick Cheney
c) Dan Quayle
d) Spiro Agnew

## Can you separate potato fact from potato fiction?

1. FACT or FICTION  Potatoes were so valued for their vitamin C content that miners traded gold for potatoes during the Klondike gold rush in1897-98.

2. FACT or FICTION  Potato chips were invented by accident.

3. FACT or FICTION  Potato leaves are poisonous.

4. FACT or FICTION  At first, the Europeans were reluctant to accept the potato because it wasn't mentioned in the Bible.

5. FACT or FICTION  The name for this popular vegetable comes from a Latin word meaning "knobby roots."

**Bonus question:**
What do Tom Brokaw, Walter Cronkite, Chet Huntley and David Brinkley have in common?

Answers on page 59

# Meet the author, the artist & the poet

**Hank Bruce** is a writer, horticultural therapist, hunger activist, teacher and speaker. He is the former president of the Florida Chapter of the American Horticultural Therapy Association. Hank has conducted research on the use of plants, flowers and gardening activities as therapeutic tools with stroke and Alzheimer's patients, and the value of gardening activities in the treatment of victims of domestic violence and substance abuse. In April 2007 he was awarded the Lifetime Achievement Award by the Florida Chapter of the American Horticultural Therapy Association and in 2001 he was given the Humanitarian of the Year Award by the American Horticultural Therapy Association. Hank's book, *Peace Beyond All Fear, a Tribute to John Denver's Vision* won the 2008 New Mexico Book of the Year Award in the anthology category. Hank & his wife Tomi have over 20 other books in print dealing with horticultural therapy, hunger issues and fiction.

**Sally Lamas**, the illustrator, offers her artistic skills for the benefit and enjoyment of her elders. Everywhere she's lived, Sally has been enriched by collaboration and companionship with extraordinary people from an array of cultures, ages and abilities. These include villagers cultivating soybeans in Mali, West Africa where she served as a Peace Corps volunteer; summer camp kids backpacking beside her in the mountains of Santa Fe, NM; teenagers maintaining open space trails in Denver, CO; men in their early twenties fighting fires on Hot Shot crews out of Grants, NM; greenhouse workers living fulfilling lives with developmental disabilities in Albuquerque, NM; and nursery employees growing plants while taming and transforming the lions of mental illnesses in San Luis Obispo, CA.

**Tomi Jill Folk**, the editor and poet, holds a Master of Divinity degree and was a pastor in Minnesota and South Dakota before the late onset of type 1 diabetes. She is now a photographer, poet, storyteller, speaker, writer and editor. She is also one of the founders and the president of the board of directors for Hunger Grow Away, a non-profit food security organization that promotes family vegetable gardens as a way to fight hunger, improve nutrition and control the spread of diabetes and heart disease. She works with many in the Native American communities in the Southwest, learning and sharing wisdom and information, hearing and telling stories. Her style is not to lecture but to listen. Her book *Visits with the Old Indian Storyteller* was a finalist in the New Mexico Book of the Year competition in 2008. In October 2008 Tomi & her husband, Hank Bruce, were honored with a Distinguished Merit award by the Northern California Council of Activity Coordinators for service and dedication to the activity profession through their publishing house Petals & Pages Press.

To read more about Hank and Tomi's work, see www.hungergrowaway.org and www.petalsandpagespress.com

## *Answers to Mashed Potato Quiz:*

*Part 1: 1. d, 2. c, 3. d, 4a, 5. a,b,c,d, 6. a, 7. b, 8. d, 9. c, 10. b, 11. d, 12. c, Part 2: 1. Fact, 2. Fact, 3. Fact, 4.Fact, 5. Fiction*

Oh, almost forgot the bonus question. *They all became **common taters.***

LaVergne, TN USA
04 December 2009
165843LV00004B/4/P